DIABETIC DIET
AFTER 50

1800+ Days of Easy, Delicious & Time-Saving Recipes for Effective Management of Type 2 Diabetes, Prediabetes, and New Diagnoses | Includes a 4-Week Meal Plan & Expert Advice

THOMAS DHARMAN

TABLE OF CONTENTS

INTRODUCTION

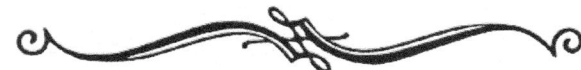

Hey there, fellow health enthusiasts and curious minds! Welcome to a journey where we dive deep into the world of diabetes and discover the power of food in managing this condition. Buckle up, because we're about to embark on a rollercoaster ride filled with eye-opening facts, practical tips, and mouthwatering recipes that'll make your taste buds dance with delight!

Let's Talk Diabetes

Alright, let's get real for a moment. Diabetes isn't just a word thrown around in medical textbooks; it's a real-life challenge faced by millions worldwide. Imagine your body playing a game of hide-and-seek with insulin, the blood sugar gatekeeper. Sometimes, it's a smooth ride, and other times, it feels like your body's throwing a rebellious tantrum. But fear not, because knowledge is power, and we're here to arm you with the tools you need to take charge of your health.

The Shocking Truth

Here's a jaw-dropping fact to kick things off: Did you know that over 400 million people are living with diabetes globally? Yep, you read that right—400 million! That's like the entire population of the United States, Canada, and Australia combined. Now, if that doesn't make you sit up and pay attention, I don't know what will!

Meet Insulin: The Unsung Hero

Let's give a round of applause to insulin, the unsung hero in our body's metabolic orchestra. Picture insulin as the conductor, orchestrating the smooth flow of glucose into our cells, where it's transformed into energy. But here's the kicker: when insulin doesn't do its job properly, chaos ensues, and blood sugar levels go haywire. It's like a symphony gone wrong—a recipe for disaster if left unchecked.

Types of Diabetes: A Crash Course

Now, let's break it down Barney-style. We've got Type 1 diabetes, the OG disruptor that throws a curveball by attacking the body's insulin-producing cells. Then there's Type 2 diabetes, the sneaky ninja that creeps up on you when you least expect it, often due to lifestyle factors like diet and exercise. Oh, and let's not forget about gestational diabetes—the unexpected plot twist that catches moms-to-be off guard during pregnancy. Yep, diabetes comes in all shapes and sizes, but armed with knowledge, we're ready to tackle it head-on.

Symptoms: Listen to Your Body's SOS Signals

Your body has a knack for sending out SOS signals when something's amiss. So, listen up! Frequent trips to the bathroom, unquenchable thirst, sudden weight loss—these are just a few red flags that your body might be waving in your face. Ignoring them is like hitting the snooze button on a fire alarm—you're only delaying the inevitable.

The Risky Business of Risk Factors

Alright, time for a reality check. While genetics certainly play a role in the diabetes game, lifestyle factors like diet and physical activity hold the winning cards. Picture this: a deck stacked with sugary snacks, sedentary lifestyles, and stress—recipe for disaster, right? But fear not, because knowledge is power, and armed with the right information, we can shuffle the deck and deal ourselves a winning hand.

Diagnosis: The Plot Thickens

Ever heard the saying, "Knowledge is power"? Well, when it comes to diabetes, early detection is your secret weapon. Enter the world of diagnostic tests—finger pricks, glucose tolerance tests, and A1C checks. It's like playing detective, uncovering clues to crack the case of unruly blood sugar levels. The sooner we catch diabetes in the act, the better equipped we are to fight back and reclaim control of our health.

What is Diabetes?

Alright, let's break it down to the basics. Diabetes isn't just a one-size-fits-all condition; it's more like a complex puzzle with many pieces. At its core, diabetes is a metabolic disorder that disrupts the body's ability to regulate blood sugar levels effectively. You see, when we eat, our bodies break down food into glucose, a fancy term for sugar. Now, normally, insulin—the body's VIP hormone—steps in to escort glucose into our cells, where it's used for energy. But in people with diabetes, this process hits a snag. Either the body doesn't produce enough insulin (Type 1 diabetes), or it becomes resistant to insulin's charms (Type 2 diabetes). The end result? A buildup of sugar in the bloodstream, wreaking havoc on our health if left unchecked.

Explanation of Insulin and its Role

Ah, insulin—the unsung hero in our body's metabolic symphony. Think of insulin as the key that unlocks the door to our cells, allowing glucose to enter and fuel our bodies. But here's the plot twist: in people with Type 1 diabetes, the body's immune system goes rogue, launching an all-out attack on the pancreas— the organ responsible for producing insulin. It's like trying to start a car with a missing key—no matter how hard you try, it's just not gonna work. On the flip side, Type 2 diabetes is more like a case of "key overload." You've got plenty of insulin floating around, but the cells have become resistant to its charms, leaving sugar stranded in the bloodstream. It's a delicate dance between supply and demand, and when the balance is thrown off, chaos ensues.

Different Types of Diabetes (Type 1, Type 2, Gestational)

Alright, let's play a game of diabetes bingo! We've got Type 1, Type 2, and gestational diabetes—three unique flavors of the same condition. Type 1 diabetes, often diagnosed in childhood or adolescence, is like getting a surprise visit from the body's immune system, which decides to wage war on the pancreas. It's an all-out battle that leaves the body's insulin production in shambles. On the other hand, Type 2 diabetes is more like a slow burn—a result of years of poor dietary choices, sedentary lifestyles, and genetic predisposition. It's the silent ninja that sneaks up on you when you least expect it, demanding attention when it's least convenient. And then there's gestational diabetes, the unexpected plot twist that catches moms-to-be off guard during pregnancy. It's like a curveball thrown into the mix, requiring extra vigilance and care to ensure a healthy outcome for both mom and baby.

Common Symptoms

Alright, time to play symptom sleuth! When it comes to diabetes, our bodies have a way of sounding the alarm when something's amiss. Think frequent trips to the bathroom, unquenchable thirst, sudden weight loss—your body's way of saying, "Houston, we have a problem!" But here's the kicker: these symptoms can be sneaky, often flying under the radar until they reach a boiling point. That's why it's essential to listen to your body's SOS signals and seek medical attention if something feels off. Ignoring the warning signs is like playing a game of chicken with your health—you're only setting yourself up for a crash landing.

Causes And Risk Factors for Diabetes and Prediabetes in Individuals Over 50

1. **Age**: As individuals age, the risk of developing diabetes significantly increases. This phenomenon is primarily due to several physiological changes that occur in the body over the years. One of these changes is the reduced capacity of the pancreas to secrete insulin in response to blood glucose. Pancreatic beta cells, responsible for insulin production, may become less efficient over time, making it more challenging for the body to maintain blood glucose regulation. Additionally, with age, cells in the body may become less sensitive to insulin action, leading to a condition known as insulin resistance. These physiological changes significantly increase the risk of developing type 2 diabetes, the most common type of diabetes in adults over 50.

2. **Obesity and Overweight**: Obesity and overweight are strong risk factors for the development of type 2 diabetes and prediabetes. Excess adipose tissue, especially in the abdominal region, is associated with chronic inflammation and increased production of hormones that can interfere with blood glucose regulation. Additionally, visceral fat may release harmful chemicals called adipokines, which can contribute to insulin resistance and systemic inflammation. Obese or overweight individuals often have higher levels of blood sugar and insulin than people of normal weight, increasing their risk of developing diabetes over time.

3. **Sedentary Lifestyle**: Insufficient physical activity is a well-known risk factor for diabetes and prediabetes. Regular exercise not only helps maintain a healthy body weight but also improves insulin sensitivity and the body's ability to utilize glucose as an energy source. Individuals who spend most of their time inactive have a higher risk of developing insulin resistance and diabetes compared to those who engage in regular physical activity. Moreover, exercise can help reduce stress, improve mood, and promote quality sleep, all of which can positively influence blood glucose regulation.

4. **Genetic Predisposition**: Genetics play a significant role in susceptibility to type 2 diabetes and prediabetes. If one or both parents have a history of diabetes, the risk of developing the disease increases significantly. However, it's essential to emphasize that genetics is not destiny. Even with a genetic predisposition to diabetes, a healthy lifestyle can significantly reduce the risk of developing the disease or delay its onset.

5. **Poor Diet**: A diet rich in added sugars, refined carbohydrates, saturated fats, and high-calorie foods can negatively affect blood glucose regulation and insulin sensitivity. Excessive consumption of high-glycemic index foods can lead to blood sugar spikes followed by sudden crashes, putting strain on the pancreas to maintain blood glucose balance over time. Additionally, a diet high in

processed and nutrient-poor foods can contribute to weight gain and inflammation, both of which are risk factors for diabetes and prediabetes.

A thorough understanding of these risk factors can help individuals over 50 make informed decisions to reduce their risk of developing diabetes or prediabetes and promote overall health through healthy lifestyle choices. Always consult a healthcare professional for a personalized risk assessment and to develop an appropriate prevention or management plan.

Appropriate Diet for a Diabetic Over 50 Years Old:

A well-balanced diet is crucial for managing diabetes effectively, especially for individuals over 50 years old. Here's a guideline for a suitable diet:

1. Control Carbohydrate Intake:

- Focus on consuming carbohydrates with a low glycemic index (GI), such as whole grains, legumes, non-starchy vegetables, and fruits.
- Limit refined carbohydrates and sugary foods, such as white bread, white rice, pastries, sugary beverages, and sweets, as they can cause rapid spikes in blood sugar levels.

2. Include Lean Proteins:

- Incorporate lean protein sources into meals, such as poultry without skin, fish, tofu, legumes, and low-fat dairy products.
- Protein helps to stabilize blood sugar levels and promotes satiety.

3. Healthy Fats:

- Choose healthy fats, such as those found in nuts, seeds, avocados, olive oil, and fatty fish like salmon and mackerel.
- Limit saturated and trans fats found in fried foods, processed snacks, and fatty cuts of meat, as they can increase the risk of heart disease.

4. Portion Control:

- Practice portion control to manage calorie intake and prevent weight gain, which is important for controlling blood sugar levels.
- Use smaller plates and bowls, and avoid going back for second helpings.

5. Emphasize Fiber-Rich Foods:

- Include plenty of fiber-rich foods in the diet, such as whole grains, fruits, vegetables, legumes, and nuts.

Fiber helps to regulate blood sugar levels, improve digestion, and promote heart health

7. Stay Hydrated:

- Drink plenty of water throughout the day to stay hydrated and support overall health.
- Limit consumption of sugary beverages and alcohol, which can contribute to blood sugar spikes and dehydration.

8. Regular Meal Timing:

- Aim for regular meal timing and spacing meals evenly throughout the day to help maintain stable blood sugar levels.
- Avoid skipping meals, as this can lead to fluctuations in blood sugar levels.

9. Monitor Blood Sugar Levels:

- Monitor blood sugar levels regularly, as dietary adjustments may be necessary based on individual blood sugar readings.
- Work closely with a healthcare provider or dietitian to develop a personalized meal plan tailored to individual needs and preferences.

By following these dietary guidelines, individuals with diabetes over 50 years old can better manage their condition, improve blood sugar control, and reduce the risk of complications associated with diabetes.

Diagnosing Diabetes

Early diagnosis of diabetes is not just about identifying symptoms—it's a critical step towards preventing complications, improving outcomes, and enhancing quality of life. Recognizing the subtleties of blood sugar regulation, understanding the nuances of diagnostic testing, and appreciating the significance of early intervention are essential components of diabetes diagnosis and management.

Blood Sugar Levels and Testing

Blood sugar levels serve as a window into the body's metabolic health, offering invaluable insights into glucose regulation and diabetes risk. Understanding the intricacies of blood sugar dynamics—both fasting and postprandial—is essential for accurate diagnosis and personalized treatment strategies. Fasting blood glucose (FBG) measurements, obtained after an overnight fast, provide a snapshot of baseline glucose levels, with values $\geq$126 mg/dL (7.0 mmol/L) indicative of diabetes. Postprandial glucose (PPG) readings, obtained after meals, reveal the body's ability to process and metabolize dietary carbohydrates, offering additional context for diabetes diagnosis and management. Hemoglobin A1C (HbA1C) testing—a gold standard in diabetes care—provides a comprehensive assessment of average blood glucose levels over the preceding 2-3 months, reflecting long-term glycemic control. Diagnostic thresholds for diabetes, established by leading medical organizations, underscore the importance of targeted interventions and personalized treatment plans based on individualized risk profiles.

Importance of Early Detection

The importance of early detection in diabetes cannot be overstated—it's a game-changer with far-reaching implications for health outcomes and quality of life. Delaying diagnosis not only increases the risk of diabetes-related complications but also limits the effectiveness of interventions aimed at preventing disease progression. Research indicates that individuals with undiagnosed diabetes are at significantly higher risk of cardiovascular disease, kidney disease, neuropathy, and retinopathy—complications that can have profound implications for morbidity and mortality. By identifying diabetes early, healthcare providers can implement timely interventions, empower patients with knowledge and resources, and foster proactive management strategies that mitigate risk and optimize long-term health outcomes.

Diagnostic Tests

A myriad of diagnostic tests are available for evaluating blood sugar levels, assessing glycemic control, and diagnosing diabetes with precision and accuracy. Fasting plasma glucose (FPG) testing, considered a cornerstone of diabetes diagnosis, involves measuring blood glucose levels after an overnight fast, with diagnostic criteria for diabetes set at FPG levels $\geq$126 mg/dL (7.0 mmol/L). Oral glucose tolerance tests

(OGTT) offer a comprehensive evaluation of glucose metabolism by measuring blood glucose levels before and after ingesting a standardized glucose solution, with diagnostic thresholds for diabetes established at 2-hour plasma glucose levels ≥200 mg/dL (11.1 mmol/L). Hemoglobin A1C (HbA1C) testing, a widely utilized tool in diabetes care, provides a holistic assessment of average blood glucose levels over a prolonged period, enabling clinicians to gauge long-term glycemic control and tailor treatment plans accordingly. Point-of-care testing (POCT) devices and continuous glucose monitoring (CGM) systems offer rapid, convenient, and real-time monitoring of blood glucose levels, facilitating timely diagnosis, treatment optimization, and proactive management of diabetes.

CHAPTER 1
BREAKFAST IDEAS

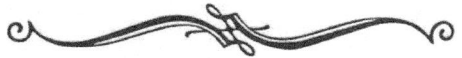

VEGGIE OMELETTE

Servings: 2
Ingredients:
- 4 large eggs
- 1/4 cup diced bell peppers
- 1/4 cup diced onions
- 1/4 cup diced tomatoes
- 1/4 cup chopped spinach
- Salt and pepper to taste

Prep Time: 5 minutes
Cook Time: 10 minutes
Instructions:
- In a bowl, whisk together the eggs until well beaten. Season with salt and pepper.
- Heat a non-stick skillet over medium heat and lightly coat with cooking spray.
- Add the diced vegetables to the skillet and sauté until tender, about 3-4 minutes.
- Pour the beaten eggs over the sautéed vegetables in the skillet.
- Cook the omelette for 3-4 minutes, or until the edges begin to set.
- Carefully flip the omelette and cook for an additional 2-3 minutes, or until cooked through.
- Serve hot with a side of whole grain toast or fresh fruit.

Nutritional Values (per serving):
- Total Carbohydrate: 5g
- Dietary Fiber: 1g
- Total Sugars: 2g
- Protein: 14g
- Total Fat: 10g
- Saturated Fat: 3g
- Cholesterol: 372mg
- Vitamin A: 1230IU
- Vitamin C: 27mg
- Folate: 96mcg
- Sodium: 376mg
- Calcium: 68mg
- Iron: 2mg
- Magnesium: 25mg
- Potassium: 330mg

GREEK YOGURT PARFAIT

Servings: 2
Ingredients:
- 1 cup plain Greek yogurt
- 1/2 cup fresh berries (such as strawberries, blueberries, or raspberries)
- 2 tablespoons chopped nuts (such as almonds or walnuts)
- 1 tablespoon honey or sugar-free sweetener (optional)

Prep Time: 5 minutes
Cook Time: 0 minutes
Instructions:
- In two serving glasses or bowls, layer the Greek yogurt, fresh berries, and chopped nuts.
- Drizzle with honey or a sugar-free sweetener if desired.
- Serve immediately or refrigerate until ready to enjoy.

Nutritional Values (per serving):
- Total Carbohydrate: 15g
- Dietary Fiber: 3g
- Total Sugars: 11g
- Protein: 15g
- Total Fat: 9g
- Saturated Fat: 1g
- Cholesterol: 10mg
- Vitamin A: 0IU
- Vitamin C: 12mg
- Folate: 9mcg
- Sodium: 56mg
- Calcium: 174mg
- Iron: 1mg
- Magnesium: 43mg
- Potassium: 250mg

AVOCADO TOAST

Servings: 2
Ingredients:
- 2 slices whole grain bread, toasted
- 1 ripe avocado, mashed
- 1 teaspoon lemon juice
- Salt and pepper to taste
- Red pepper flakes (optional)

Prep Time: 5 minutes
Cook Time: 0 minutes
Instructions:
- In a bowl, mash the ripe avocado with lemon juice until smooth.
- Season the mashed avocado with salt, pepper, and red pepper flakes if desired.
- Spread the mashed avocado evenly onto the toasted whole grain bread slices.
- Serve immediately.

Nutritional Values (per serving):
- Total Carbohydrate: 24g
- Dietary Fiber: 10g
- Total Sugars: 1g
- Protein: 6g
- Total Fat: 15g
- Saturated Fat: 2g
- Cholesterol: 0mg
- Vitamin A: 82IU
- Vitamin C: 11mg
- Folate: 111mcg
- Sodium: 175mg
- Calcium: 35mg
- Iron: 1mg
- Magnesium: 29mg
- Potassium: 490mg

QUINOA BREAKFAST BOWL

Servings: 2
Ingredients:
- 1/2 cup quinoa, rinsed
- 1 cup water or low-sodium vegetable broth
- 1/2 teaspoon ground cinnamon
- 1/4 cup chopped nuts (such as almonds or pecans)
- 1/4 cup fresh berries (such as strawberries or blueberries)
- 2 tablespoons Greek yogurt
- 1 tablespoon honey or sugar-free sweetener (optional)

Prep Time: 5 minutes
Cook Time: 15 minutes
Instructions:
- In a small saucepan, combine the quinoa and water or broth. Bring to a boil, then reduce heat to low, cover, and simmer for 12-15 minutes, or until the quinoa is tender and the liquid is absorbed.
- Stir in the ground cinnamon.
- Divide the cooked quinoa into two bowls.
- Top each bowl with chopped nuts, fresh berries, Greek yogurt, and a drizzle of honey or sugar-free sweetener if desired.
- Serve warm.

Nutritional Values (per serving):
- Total Carbohydrate: 35g
- Dietary Fiber: 5g
- Total Sugars: 10g
- Protein: 10g
- Total Fat: 8g
- Saturated Fat: 1g
- Cholesterol: 1mg
- Vitamin A: 30IU
- Vitamin C: 2mg
- Folate: 75mcg
- Sodium: 5mg
- Calcium: 48mg
- Iron: 2mg
- Magnesium: 91mg
- Potassium: 239mg

SPINACH AND FETA EGG MUFFINS

Servings: 4
Ingredients:
- 6 large eggs
- 1 cup chopped spinach
- 1/4 cup crumbled feta cheese
- 1/4 cup diced tomatoes
- Salt and pepper to taste

Prep Time: 10 minutes
Cook Time: 20 minutes
Instructions:
- Preheat the oven to 350°F (175°C). Grease a muffin tin or line with silicone muffin liners.
- In a large mixing bowl, whisk together the eggs until well beaten. Season with salt and pepper.
- Stir in the chopped spinach, crumbled feta cheese, and diced tomatoes until evenly combined.
- Pour the egg mixture into the prepared muffin tin, filling each cup about 3/4 full.
- Bake in the preheated oven for 18-20 minutes, or until the egg muffins are set and lightly golden on top.
- Allow the egg muffins to cool slightly before serving.

Nutritional Values (per serving):
- Total Carbohydrate: 2g
- Dietary Fiber: 1g
- Total Sugars: 1g
- Protein: 11g
- Total Fat: 6g
- Saturated Fat: 2g
- Cholesterol: 240mg
- Vitamin A: 855IU
- Vitamin C: 3mg
- Folate: 52mcg
- Sodium: 249mg
- Calcium: 86mg
- Iron: 1mg
- Magnesium: 20mg
- Potassium: 147mg

BERRY CHIA SEED PUDDING

Servings: 2
Ingredients:
- 1/4 cup chia seeds
- 1 cup unsweetened almond milk
- 1/2 teaspoon vanilla extract
- 1/2 cup fresh berries (such as strawberries or raspberries)
- 1 tablespoon chopped nuts (such as almonds or walnuts)
- 1 tablespoon unsweetened shredded coconut (optional)

Prep Time: 5 minutes
Cook Time: 0 minutes (plus refrigeration time)
Instructions:
- In a mixing bowl, combine the chia seeds, almond milk, and vanilla extract. Stir well to combine.
- Cover the bowl and refrigerate for at least 2 hours, or until the chia seeds have absorbed the liquid and the mixture has thickened to a pudding-like consistency.
- Once the chia pudding is set, divide it into two serving bowls.
- Top each bowl with fresh berries, chopped nuts, and shredded coconut if desired.
- Serve chilled.

Nutritional Values (per serving):
- Total Carbohydrate: 15g
- Dietary Fiber: 10g
- Total Sugars: 3g
- Protein: 5g
- Total Fat: 10g
- Saturated Fat: 1g
- Cholesterol: 0mg
- Vitamin A: 0IU
- Vitamin C: 13mg
- Folate: 36mcg
- Sodium: 84mg
- Calcium: 289mg
- Iron: 2mg
- Magnesium: 93mg
- Potassium: 161mg

WHOLE GRAIN PANCAKES

Servings: 4
Ingredients:
- 1 cup whole wheat flour
- 1 tablespoon baking powder
- 1/4 teaspoon salt
- 1 tablespoon sugar or sugar-free sweetener
- 1 cup unsweetened almond milk
- 1 large egg
- 2 tablespoons unsweetened applesauce
- 1 teaspoon vanilla extract
- Cooking spray or oil for greasing the skillet
- Fresh fruit and sugar-free syrup for serving

Prep Time: 10 minutes
Cook Time: 10 minutes
Instructions:
- In a large mixing bowl, whisk together the whole wheat flour, baking powder, salt, and sugar or sugar-free sweetener.
- In a separate bowl, whisk together the almond milk, egg, applesauce, and vanilla extract until well combined.
- Pour the wet ingredients into the dry ingredients and stir until just combined. Do not overmix—the batter may be slightly lumpy.
- Heat a non-stick skillet or griddle over medium heat and lightly coat with cooking spray or oil.
- Pour 1/4 cup of batter onto the skillet for each pancake.
- Cook until bubbles form on the surface of the pancakes and the edges appear set, then flip and cook for an additional 1-2 minutes, or until golden brown.
- Repeat with the remaining batter.
- Serve the pancakes warm with fresh fruit and sugar-free syrup.

Nutritional Values (per serving):
- Total Carbohydrate: 25g
- Dietary Fiber: 3g
- Total Sugars: 2g
- Protein: 5g
- Total Fat: 2g
- Saturated Fat: 0g
- Cholesterol: 47mg
- Vitamin A: 56IU
- Vitamin C: 0mg
- Folate: 35mcg
- Sodium: 539mg
- Calcium: 241mg
- Iron: 1mg
- Magnesium: 33mg
- Potassium: 123mg

BANANA NUT OVERNIGHT OATS

Servings: 2
Ingredients:
- 1 cup old-fashioned rolled oats
- 1 cup unsweetened almond milk
- 1 ripe banana, mashed
- 2 tablespoons chopped nuts (such as walnuts or pecans)
- 1 tablespoon chia seeds
- 1/2 teaspoon ground cinnamon
- 1 tablespoon honey or sugar-free sweetener (optional)

Prep Time: 5 minutes (plus refrigeration time)
Cook Time: 0 minutes
Instructions:
- In a mixing bowl or jar, combine the rolled oats, almond milk, mashed banana, chopped nuts, chia seeds, ground cinnamon, and honey or sugar-free sweetener if desired. Stir well to combine.
- Cover the bowl or jar and refrigerate overnight, or for at least 4 hours, to allow the oats to soften and absorb the liquid.
- Once the overnight oats are set, stir well before serving.
- Divide the oats into two serving bowls and top with additional chopped nuts or fresh fruit if desired.
- Serve chilled.

Nutritional Values (per serving):
- Total Carbohydrate: 39g
- Dietary Fiber: 7g
- Total Sugars: 10g
- Protein: 7g
- Total Fat: 9g
- Saturated Fat: 1g
- Cholesterol: 0mg
- Vitamin A: 49IU
- Vitamin C: 5mg

- Folate: 30mcg
- Sodium: 90mg
- Calcium: 179mg
- Iron: 2mg
- Magnesium: 105mg
- Potassium: 305mg

TOFU SCRAMBLE

Servings: 2
Ingredients:
- 1 tablespoon olive oil
- 1/2 cup diced bell peppers
- 1/4 cup diced onions
- 1 cup diced firm tofu
- 1/2 teaspoon ground turmeric
- Salt and pepper to taste
- 2 tablespoons nutritional yeast (optional)

Prep Time: 10 minutes
Cook Time: 10 minutes
Instructions:
- Heat olive oil in a skillet over medium heat.
- Add diced bell peppers and onions to the skillet and sauté until softened, about 3-4 minutes.
- Crumble the firm tofu into the skillet and cook, stirring occasionally, until heated through, about 5-6 minutes.
- Season the tofu scramble with ground turmeric, salt, and pepper to taste. Stir in nutritional yeast if desired.
- Continue cooking for another 2-3 minutes, or until the flavors are well combined and the tofu is lightly browned.
- Serve hot with whole grain toast or fresh fruit on the side.

Nutritional Values (per serving):
- Total Carbohydrate: 6g
- Dietary Fiber: 2g
- Total Sugars: 2g
- Protein: 8g
- Total Fat: 6g
- Saturated Fat: 1g
- Cholesterol: 0mg
- Vitamin A: 849IU
- Vitamin C: 29mg
- Folate: 20mcg
- Sodium: 240mg
- Calcium: 54mg

- Iron: 2mg
- Magnesium: 33mg
- Potassium: 227mg

BERRY PROTEIN SMOOTHIE

Servings: 2
Ingredients:
- 1 cup unsweetened almond milk
- 1/2 cup plain Greek yogurt
- 1 cup mixed berries (such as strawberries, blueberries, and raspberries)
- 1 scoop vanilla protein powder (unsweetened or sugar-free)
- 1 tablespoon almond butter or peanut butter
- 1/2 teaspoon vanilla extract
- Ice cubes (optional)

Prep Time: 5 minutes
Cook Time: 0 minutes
Instructions:
- In a blender, combine the unsweetened almond milk, plain Greek yogurt, mixed berries, vanilla protein powder, almond butter or peanut butter, and vanilla extract.
- Add ice cubes if desired for a thicker consistency.
- Blend until smooth and creamy.
- Divide the smoothie into two glasses and serve immediately.

Nutritional Values (per serving):
- Total Carbohydrate: 17g
- Dietary Fiber: 5g
- Total Sugars: 8g
- Protein: 20g
- Total Fat: 8g
- Saturated Fat: 1g
- Cholesterol: 10mg
- Vitamin A: 193IU
- Vitamin C: 16mg
- Folate: 23mcg
- Sodium: 178mg
- Calcium: 217mg
- Iron: 1mg
- Magnesium: 54mg
- Potassium: 332mg

PEANUT BUTTER BANANA SMOOTHIE BOWL

Servings: 2
Ingredients:
- 2 ripe bananas, frozen
- 1/4 cup natural peanut butter (unsweetened)
- 1 cup unsweetened almond milk
- 2 tablespoons unsweetened cocoa powder
- 1 tablespoon honey or sugar-free sweetener (optional)
- Toppings: sliced banana, chopped nuts, unsweetened shredded coconut (optional)

Prep Time: 5 minutes
Cook Time: 0 minutes
Instructions:
- In a blender, combine the frozen bananas, natural peanut butter, unsweetened almond milk, cocoa powder, and honey or sugar-free sweetener if desired.
- Blend until smooth and creamy.
- Pour the smoothie into two serving bowls.
- Top each bowl with sliced banana, chopped nuts, and shredded coconut if desired.
- Serve immediately.

Nutritional Values (per serving):
- Total Carbohydrate: 29g
- Dietary Fiber: 7g
- Total Sugars: 12g
- Protein: 10g
- Total Fat: 18g
- Saturated Fat: 3g
- Cholesterol: 0mg
- Vitamin A: 76IU
- Vitamin C: 8mg
- Folate: 27mcg
- Sodium: 173mg
- Calcium: 79mg
- Iron: 2mg
- Magnesium: 90mg
- Potassium: 544mg

MEDITERRANEAN BREAKFAST WRAP

Servings: 2
Ingredients:
- 2 whole wheat tortillas
- 4 large eggs
- 1/4 cup diced tomatoes
- 1/4 cup diced cucumber
- 2 tablespoons crumbled feta cheese
- 2 tablespoons chopped fresh parsley
- Salt and pepper to taste

Prep Time: 10 minutes
Cook Time: 10 minutes
Instructions:
- Heat a non-stick skillet over medium heat and lightly coat with cooking spray.
- Crack the eggs into the skillet and cook to desired doneness, either scrambled or fried.
- Season the eggs with salt and pepper to taste.
- Warm the whole wheat tortillas in the skillet or microwave until pliable.
- Divide the scrambled or fried eggs between the two tortillas.
- Top each tortilla with diced tomatoes, diced cucumber, crumbled feta cheese, and chopped fresh parsley.
- Roll up the tortillas into wraps and serve immediately.

Nutritional Values (per serving):
- Total Carbohydrate: 26g
- Dietary Fiber: 4g
- Total Sugars: 2g
- Protein: 17g
- Total Fat: 14g
- Saturated Fat: 5g
- Cholesterol: 378mg
- Vitamin A: 735IU
- Vitamin C: 12mg
- Folate: 102mcg
- Sodium: 573mg
- Calcium: 149mg
- Iron: 3mg
- Magnesium: 47mg
- Potassium: 324mg

BREAKFAST BURRITO

Servings: 2
Ingredients:
- 2 whole wheat tortillas
- 4 large eggs
- 1/4 cup diced bell peppers
- 1/4 cup diced onions
- 1/4 cup diced tomatoes
- 1/4 cup black beans, drained and rinsed
- 2 tablespoons shredded cheddar cheese
- 1 tablespoon chopped fresh cilantro
- Salt and pepper to taste

Prep Time: 10 minutes
Cook Time: 10 minutes
Instructions:
- Heat a non-stick skillet over medium heat and lightly coat with cooking spray.
- Add diced bell peppers and onions to the skillet and sauté until softened, about 3-4 minutes.
- Crack the eggs into the skillet and scramble until cooked through.
- Season the eggs with salt and pepper to taste.
- Warm the whole wheat tortillas in the skillet or microwave until pliable.
- Divide the scrambled eggs between the two tortillas.
- Top each tortilla with diced tomatoes, black beans, shredded cheddar cheese, and chopped fresh cilantro.
- Roll up the tortillas into burritos and serve immediately.

Nutritional Values (per serving):
- Total Carbohydrate: 25g
- Dietary Fiber: 6g
- Total Sugars: 3g
- Protein: 20g
- Total Fat: 16g
- Saturated Fat: 6g
- Cholesterol: 384mg
- Vitamin A: 1018IU
- Vitamin C: 30mg
- Folate: 69mcg
- Sodium: 494mg
- Calcium: 170mg
- Iron: 4mg
- Magnesium: 72mg
- Potassium: 474mg

BREAKFAST QUINOA BOWL

Servings: 2
Ingredients:
- 1/2 cup quinoa, rinsed
- 1 cup water or low-sodium vegetable broth
- 1/2 teaspoon ground cinnamon
- 1/4 cup chopped nuts (such as almonds or walnuts)
- 1/4 cup fresh berries (such as strawberries or blueberries)
- 2 tablespoons Greek yogurt
- 1 tablespoon honey or sugar-free sweetener (optional)

Prep Time: 5 minutes
Cook Time: 15 minutes
Instructions:
- In a small saucepan, combine the quinoa and water or broth. Bring to a boil, then reduce heat to low, cover, and simmer for 12-15 minutes, or until the quinoa is tender and the liquid is absorbed.
- Stir in the ground cinnamon.
- Divide the cooked quinoa into two bowls.
- Top each bowl with chopped nuts, fresh berries, Greek yogurt, and a drizzle of honey or sugar-free sweetener if desired.
- Serve warm.

Nutritional Values (per serving):
- Total Carbohydrate: 25g
- Dietary Fiber: 4g
- Total Sugars: 5g
- Protein: 8g
- Total Fat: 9g
- Saturated Fat: 1g
- Cholesterol: 5mg
- Vitamin A: 36IU
- Vitamin C: 2mg
- Folate: 46mcg
- Sodium: 7mg
- Calcium: 70mg
- Iron: 2mg
- Magnesium: 80mg
- Potassium: 239mg

VEGGIE BREAKFAST CASSEROLE

Servings: 4
Ingredients:
- 8 large eggs
- 1 cup diced bell peppers
- 1/2 cup diced onions
- 1 cup diced tomatoes
- 1 cup chopped spinach
- 1/2 cup shredded cheddar cheese
- Salt and pepper to taste

Prep Time: 10 minutes
Cook Time: 30 minutes
Instructions:
- Preheat the oven to 350°F (175°C). Grease a baking dish with cooking spray.
- In a large mixing bowl, whisk together the eggs until well beaten. Season with salt and pepper.
- Stir in the diced bell peppers, onions, tomatoes, chopped spinach, and shredded cheddar cheese until evenly combined.
- Pour the egg mixture into the prepared baking dish.
- Bake in the preheated oven for 25-30 minutes, or until the eggs are set and the top is golden brown.
- Allow the breakfast casserole to cool slightly before slicing and serving.

Nutritional Values (per serving):
- Total Carbohydrate: 9g
- Dietary Fiber: 2g
- Total Sugars: 4g
- Protein: 16g
- Total Fat: 12g
- Saturated Fat: 5g
- Cholesterol: 372mg
- Vitamin A: 1804IU
- Vitamin C: 56mg
- Folate: 99mcg
- Sodium: 346mg
- Calcium: 188mg
- Iron: 3mg
- Magnesium: 63mg
- Potassium: 464mg

CHAPTER 2
SNACKS OPTIONS

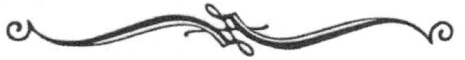

GREEK YOGURT PARFAIT

Servings: 2
Ingredients:
- 1 cup plain Greek yogurt
- 1/2 cup fresh berries (such as strawberries or blueberries)
- 1/4 cup granola (choose a low-sugar option)
- 1 tablespoon honey or sugar-free sweetener (optional)

Prep Time: 5 minutes
Cook Time: 0 minutes
Instructions:
- In two serving glasses or bowls, layer the plain Greek yogurt, fresh berries, and granola.
- Repeat the layers until the ingredients are used up.
- Drizzle honey or sugar-free sweetener over the top if desired.
- Serve immediately.

Nutritional Values (per serving):
- Total Carbohydrate: 24g
- Dietary Fiber: 3g
- Total Sugars: 12g
- Protein: 16g
- Total Fat: 4g
- Saturated Fat: 0g
- Cholesterol: 10mg
- Vitamin A: 105IU
- Vitamin C: 17mg
- Folate: 23mcg
- Sodium: 56mg
- Calcium: 197mg
- Iron: 1mg
- Magnesium: 35mg
- Potassium: 254mg

VEGGIE STICKS WITH HUMMUS

Servings: 2
Ingredients:
- 2 medium carrots, peeled and cut into sticks
- 2 celery stalks, cut into sticks
- 1/2 English cucumber, cut into sticks
- 1/2 cup hummus (choose a low-fat and low-sodium option)

Prep Time: 10 minutes
Cook Time: 0 minutes
Instructions:
- Arrange the carrot sticks, celery sticks, and cucumber sticks on a serving plate.
- Place the hummus in a small bowl in the center of the plate.
- Serve immediately.

Nutritional Values (per serving):
- Total Carbohydrate: 16g
- Dietary Fiber: 6g
- Total Sugars: 3g
- Protein: 9g
- Total Fat: 6g
- Saturated Fat: 1g
- Cholesterol: 0mg
- Vitamin A: 10111IU
- Vitamin C: 7mg
- Folate: 50mcg
- Sodium: 303mg
- Calcium: 79mg
- Iron: 2mg
- Magnesium: 24mg
- Potassium: 455mg

APPLE SLICES WITH ALMOND BUTTER

Servings: 2
Ingredients:
- 1 medium apple, sliced
- 2 tablespoons almond butter (choose a natural and unsweetened option)

Prep Time: 5 minutes
Cook Time: 0 minutes
Instructions:
- Arrange the apple slices on a serving plate.
- Serve the almond butter on the side in a small dish for dipping.
- Serve immediately.

Nutritional Values (per serving):
- Total Carbohydrate: 21g
- Dietary Fiber: 5g
- Total Sugars: 14g
- Protein: 4g
- Total Fat: 10g
- Saturated Fat: 1g
- Cholesterol: 0mg
- Vitamin A: 73IU
- Vitamin C: 8mg
- Folate: 5mcg
- Sodium: 2mg
- Calcium: 66mg
- Iron: 1mg
- Magnesium: 40mg
- Potassium: 211mg

COTTAGE CHEESE WITH PINEAPPLE

Servings: 2
Ingredients:
- 1 cup low-fat cottage cheese
- 1 cup diced pineapple (fresh or canned in its own juice)

Prep Time: 5 minutes
Cook Time: 0 minutes
Instructions:
- Divide the low-fat cottage cheese into two serving bowls.
- Top each bowl with diced pineapple.
- Serve immediately.

Nutritional Values (per serving):
- Total Carbohydrate: 24g
- Dietary Fiber: 2g
- Total Sugars: 20g
- Protein: 16g
- Total Fat: 2g
- Saturated Fat: 1g
- Cholesterol: 9mg
- Vitamin A: 113IU
- Vitamin C: 59mg
- Folate: 15mcg
- Sodium: 530mg
- Calcium: 109mg
- Iron: 1mg
- Magnesium: 29mg
- Potassium: 346mg

AVOCADO TOAST

Servings: 2
Ingredients:
- 2 slices whole grain bread, toasted
- 1 ripe avocado, mashed
- 1/2 teaspoon red pepper flakes (optional)
- Salt and pepper to taste

Prep Time: 5 minutes
Cook Time: 0 minutes
Instructions:
- Spread the mashed avocado evenly onto the toasted whole grain bread slices.
- Sprinkle with red pepper flakes if desired, and season with salt and pepper to taste.
- Serve immediately.

Nutritional Values (per serving):
Total Carbohydrate: 21g
Dietary Fiber: 7g
Total Sugars: 2g
Protein: 5g
Total Fat: 15g
Saturated Fat: 2g
Cholesterol: 0mg
Vitamin A: 121IU
Vitamin C: 10mg
Folate: 71mcg
Sodium: 202mg
Calcium: 39mg
Iron: 1mg
Magnesium: 45mg
Potassium: 487mg

EDAMAME WITH SEA SALT

Servings: 2
Ingredients:

- 1 cup cooked edamame (soybeans)
- Sea salt to taste

Prep Time: 5 minutes
Cook Time: 5 minutes (if using frozen edamame)
Instructions:

- If using frozen edamame, cook according to package instructions, then drain and set aside to cool slightly.
- Sprinkle the cooked edamame with sea salt to taste.
- Serve warm or at room temperature.

Nutritional Values (per serving):

- Total Carbohydrate: 9g
- Dietary Fiber: 4g
- Total Sugars: 2g
- Protein: 9g
- Total Fat: 3g
- Saturated Fat: 0g
- Cholesterol: 0mg
- Vitamin A: 98IU
- Vitamin C: 3mg
- Folate: 121mcg
- Sodium: 6mg
- Calcium: 52mg
- Iron: 2mg
- Magnesium: 99mg
- Potassium: 436mg

CUCUMBER ROLL-UPS

Servings: 2
Ingredients:

- 1 large cucumber
- 1/4 cup hummus (choose a low-fat and low-sodium option)
- 1/4 cup thinly sliced red bell pepper
- 1/4 cup thinly sliced carrot

Prep Time: 10 minutes
Cook Time: 0 minutes
Instructions:

- Use a vegetable peeler to slice the cucumber lengthwise into thin strips.
- Spread a thin layer of hummus onto each cucumber strip.
- Place a few slices of red bell pepper and carrot onto each cucumber strip.
- Roll up the cucumber strips tightly to form roll-ups.
- Secure with toothpicks if necessary.
- Serve immediately.

Nutritional Values (per serving):

- Total Carbohydrate: 11g
- Dietary Fiber: 3g
- Total Sugars: 4g
- Protein: 4g
- Total Fat: 3g
- Saturated Fat: 0g
- Cholesterol: 0mg
- Vitamin A: 3087IU
- Vitamin C: 28mg
- Folate: 23mcg
- Sodium: 108mg
- Calcium: 44mg
- Iron: 1mg
- Magnesium: 21mg
- Potassium: 306mg

ALMOND BERRY ENERGY BALLS

Servings: 2
Ingredients:
- 1/2 cup rolled oats
- 1/4 cup almond butter (choose a natural and unsweetened option)
- 2 tablespoons honey or maple syrup
- 1/4 cup dried berries (such as cranberries or cherries), chopped
- 2 tablespoons ground flaxseed
- 2 tablespoons unsweetened shredded coconut

Prep Time: 10 minutes
Cook Time: 0 minutes
Instructions:
- In a mixing bowl, combine the rolled oats, almond butter, honey or maple syrup, dried berries, ground flaxseed, and shredded coconut.
- Stir until the mixture is well combined and holds together when pressed.
- Roll the mixture into bite-sized balls using your hands.
- Place the energy balls on a plate or baking sheet lined with parchment paper.
- Chill in the refrigerator for at least 30 minutes to firm up.
- Serve chilled.

Nutritional Values (per serving):
- Total Carbohydrate: 29g
- Dietary Fiber: 5g
- Total Sugars: 16g
- Protein: 7g
- Total Fat: 17g
- Saturated Fat: 2g
- Cholesterol: 0mg
- Vitamin A: 1IU
- Vitamin C: 0mg
- Folate: 23mcg
- Sodium: 4mg
- Calcium: 77mg
- Iron: 2mg
- Magnesium: 85mg
- Potassium: 258mg

CAPRESE SKEWERS

Servings: 2
Ingredients:
- 8 cherry tomatoes
- 8 fresh basil leaves
- 4 small mozzarella balls (bocconcini)
- Balsamic glaze (optional)

Prep Time: 10 minutes
Cook Time: 0 minutes
Instructions:
- Thread a cherry tomato, a basil leaf, and a mozzarella ball onto each skewer.
- Arrange the skewers on a serving plate.
- Drizzle with balsamic glaze if desired.
- Serve immediately.

Nutritional Values (per serving):
- Total Carbohydrate: 6g
- Dietary Fiber: 1g
- Total Sugars: 3g
- Protein: 9g
- Total Fat: 9g
- Saturated Fat: 5g
- Cholesterol: 27mg
- Vitamin A: 597IU
- Vitamin C: 18mg
- Folate: 5mcg
- Sodium: 15mg
- Calcium: 192mg
- Iron: 1mg
- Magnesium: 8mg
- Potassium: 84mg

TURKEY AND CHEESE ROLL-UPS

Servings: 2
Ingredients:

- 4 slices deli turkey breast
- 2 slices reduced-fat cheese (such as cheddar or Swiss)
- 1/4 cup baby spinach leaves

Prep Time: 5 minutes
Cook Time: 0 minutes
Instructions:

- Lay out the turkey slices on a flat surface.
- Place a slice of cheese on each turkey slice.
- Top each slice with baby spinach leaves.
- Roll up the turkey slices tightly to form roll-ups.
- Secure with toothpicks if necessary.
- Serve immediately.

Nutritional Values (per serving):

- Total Carbohydrate: 3g
- Dietary Fiber: 0g
- Total Sugars: 1g
- Protein: 15g
- Total Fat: 7g
- Saturated Fat: 2g
- Cholesterol: 52mg
- Vitamin A: 571IU
- Vitamin C: 2mg
- Folate: 8mcg
- Sodium: 391mg
- Calcium: 179mg
- Iron: 1mg
- Magnesium: 15mg
- Potassium: 239mg

CHAPTER 3
VEGETARIAN MAINS LOW-CARB AND HIGH-FIBER RECIPES

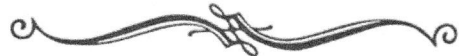

ZUCCHINI NOODLES WITH PESTO

Servings: 2
Ingredients:
- 2 medium zucchini
- 1/4 cup prepared pesto sauce (choose a low-carb and low-sodium option)
- 1/4 cup cherry tomatoes, halved
- 2 tablespoons grated Parmesan cheese (optional)

Prep Time: 10 minutes
Cook Time: 5 minutes
Instructions:
- Use a spiralizer to create zucchini noodles from the zucchini or use a vegetable peeler to make ribbons.
- Heat a non-stick skillet over medium heat and add the zucchini noodles. Cook for 2-3 minutes until just tender.
- Toss the cooked zucchini noodles with the pesto sauce until evenly coated.
- Divide the zucchini noodles between two serving plates and top with cherry tomatoes and grated Parmesan cheese if desired.
- Serve immediately.

Nutritional Values (per serving):
- Total Carbohydrate: 9g
- Dietary Fiber: 3g
- Total Sugars: 5g
- Protein: 4g
- Total Fat: 16g
- Saturated Fat: 3g
- Cholesterol: 6mg
- Vitamin A: 833IU
- Vitamin C: 35mg
- Folate: 35mcg
- Sodium: 175mg
- Calcium: 119mg
- Iron: 1mg

- Magnesium: 48mg
- Potassium: 512mg

CAULIFLOWER FRIED RICE

Servings: 2
Ingredients:
- 2 cups cauliflower rice (fresh or frozen)
- 1/4 cup diced carrots
- 1/4 cup diced bell peppers
- 1/4 cup diced onions
- 2 cloves garlic, minced
- 2 tablespoons low-sodium soy sauce or tamari
- 1 tablespoon sesame oil
- 2 eggs, beaten
- 2 green onions, thinly sliced

Prep Time: 10 minutes
Cook Time: 10 minutes
Instructions:
- Heat the sesame oil in a large skillet or wok over medium heat.
- Add the diced carrots, bell peppers, onions, and garlic to the skillet. Cook for 3-4 minutes until softened.
- Push the vegetables to one side of the skillet and pour the beaten eggs into the empty space. Scramble the eggs until cooked through, then mix with the cooked vegetables.
- Add the cauliflower rice and low-sodium soy sauce to the skillet. Stir well to combine.
- Cook for another 3-4 minutes until the cauliflower rice is heated through.
- Remove from heat and stir in the sliced green onions.
- Serve hot.

Nutritional Values (per serving):
- Total Carbohydrate: 14g
- Dietary Fiber: 5g
- Total Sugars: 6g
- Protein: 9g

- Total Fat: 11g
- Saturated Fat: 2g
- Cholesterol: 186mg
- Vitamin A: 4275IU
- Vitamin C: 102mg
- Folate: 89mcg
- Sodium: 641mg
- Calcium: 107mg
- Iron: 2mg
- Magnesium: 34mg
- Potassium: 538mg

LENTIL AND VEGETABLE CURRY

Servings: 4
Ingredients:
- 1 cup dried green lentils, rinsed and drained
- 1 tablespoon olive oil
- 1 onion, diced
- 2 cloves garlic, minced
- 1 tablespoon grated ginger
- 1 tablespoon curry powder
- 1 teaspoon ground turmeric
- 1 can (14 oz) diced tomatoes
- 1 can (14 oz) coconut milk
- 2 cups chopped mixed vegetables (such as bell peppers, carrots, and spinach)
- Salt and pepper to taste

Prep Time: 10 minutes
Cook Time: 30 minutes
Instructions:
- In a large pot, heat the olive oil over medium heat. Add the diced onion and cook until softened, about 5 minutes.
- Add the minced garlic, grated ginger, curry powder, and ground turmeric to the pot. Cook for another 2 minutes until fragrant.
- Stir in the diced tomatoes (with their juices), coconut milk, and rinsed lentils. Bring to a simmer.
- Cover and cook for 20-25 minutes, stirring occasionally, until the lentils are tender.
- Add the chopped mixed vegetables to the pot and continue to cook for another 5 minutes until the vegetables are tender.
- Season with salt and pepper to taste.
- Serve hot, optionally with rice or naan bread.

Nutritional Values (per serving):
- Total Carbohydrate: 35g
- Dietary Fiber: 10g
- Total Sugars: 8g
- Protein: 13g
- Total Fat: 14g
- Saturated Fat: 9g
- Cholesterol: 0mg
- Vitamin A: 3615IU
- Vitamin C: 29mg
- Folate: 242mcg
- Sodium: 25mg
- Calcium: 98mg
- Iron: 5mg
- Magnesium: 92mg
- Potassium: 741mg

PORTOBELLO MUSHROOM BURGERS

Servings: 2
Ingredients:
- 2 large portobello mushroom caps
- 2 whole grain burger buns
- 1/4 cup balsamic vinegar
- 2 tablespoons olive oil
- 2 cloves garlic, minced
- 1 teaspoon dried thyme
- Salt and pepper to taste
- Toppings: lettuce, tomato slices, avocado slices (optional)

Prep Time: 10 minutes
Cook Time: 10 minutes
Instructions:
- In a small bowl, whisk together the balsamic vinegar, olive oil, minced garlic, dried thyme, salt, and pepper.
- Place the portobello mushroom caps in a shallow dish and pour the marinade over them. Let marinate for at least 30 minutes, flipping halfway through.
- Preheat the grill or a grill pan over medium heat. Remove the mushrooms from the marinade and grill for 4-5 minutes per side, until tender.
- Toast the whole grain burger buns on the grill for 1-2 minutes.
- Assemble the burgers by placing the grilled portobello mushroom caps on the toasted buns.

Add your desired toppings such as lettuce, tomato slices, and avocado slices.
- Serve hot.

Nutritional Values (per serving):
- Total Carbohydrate: 39g
- Dietary Fiber: 8g
- Total Sugars: 10g
- Protein: 12g
- Total Fat: 16g
- Saturated Fat: 2g
- Cholesterol: 0mg
- Vitamin A: 4IU
- Vitamin C: 2mg
- Folate: 116mcg
- Sodium: 205mg
- Calcium: 92mg
- Iron: 3mg
- Magnesium: 35mg
- Potassium: 886mg

SPINACH AND FETA STUFFED PEPPERS

Servings: 2
Ingredients:
- 2 large bell peppers, halved and seeded
- 2 cups fresh spinach leaves
- 1/2 cup crumbled feta cheese
- 1/4 cup diced tomatoes
- 2 cloves garlic, minced
- 1/4 teaspoon dried oregano
- Salt and pepper to taste

Prep Time: 15 minutes
Cook Time: 25 minutes
Instructions:
- Preheat the oven to 375°F (190°C). Place the bell pepper halves in a baking dish, cut side up.
- In a skillet, wilt the spinach over medium heat for 2-3 minutes. Drain any excess liquid.
- In a mixing bowl, combine the wilted spinach, crumbled feta cheese, diced tomatoes, minced garlic, dried oregano, salt, and pepper.
- Stuff the bell pepper halves with the spinach and feta mixture.
- Cover the baking dish with foil and bake in the preheated oven for 20 minutes.
- Remove the foil and bake for an additional 5 minutes, or until the peppers are tender and the filling is heated through.
- Serve hot.

Nutritional Values (per serving):
- Total Carbohydrate: 14g
- Dietary Fiber: 5g
- Total Sugars: 8g
- Protein: 10g
- Total Fat: 7g
- Saturated Fat: 4g
- Cholesterol: 25mg
- Vitamin A: 5616IU
- Vitamin C: 186mg
- Folate: 183mcg
- Sodium: 487mg
- Calcium: 258mg
- Iron: 4mg
- Magnesium: 69mg
- Potassium: 723mg

EGGPLANT PARMESAN

Servings: 4
Ingredients:
- 1 large eggplant, sliced into 1/2-inch rounds
- 1 cup marinara sauce (choose a low-sugar option)
- 1 cup shredded mozzarella cheese
- 1/4 cup grated Parmesan cheese
- 1/4 cup breadcrumbs (optional, use almond flour for a low-carb alternative)
- 1 teaspoon dried Italian seasoning
- Salt and pepper to taste

Prep Time: 15 minutes
Cook Time: 25 minutes
Instructions:
- Preheat the oven to 375°F (190°C). Line a baking sheet with parchment paper.
- Arrange the eggplant slices on the prepared baking sheet. Season with salt and pepper.
- Bake in the preheated oven for 15 minutes, flipping halfway through, until tender.
- Remove the eggplant slices from the oven and top each slice with marinara sauce, shredded mozzarella cheese, and grated Parmesan cheese.
- In a small bowl, mix the breadcrumbs (or almond flour) with dried Italian seasoning. Sprinkle over the cheese.

- Return to the oven and bake for another 10 minutes, or until the cheese is melted and bubbly.
- Serve hot, optionally garnished with fresh basil.

Nutritional Values (per serving):
- Total Carbohydrate: 15g
- Dietary Fiber: 6g
- Total Sugars: 7g
- Protein: 11g
- Total Fat: 9g
- Saturated Fat: 5g
- Cholesterol: 30mg
- Vitamin A: 908IU
- Vitamin C: 7mg
- Folate: 42mcg
- Sodium: 632mg
- Calcium: 245mg
- Iron: 1mg
- Magnesium: 28mg
- Potassium: 372mg

SPAGHETTI SQUASH WITH TOMATO BASIL SAUCE

Servings: 2
Ingredients:
- 1 medium spaghetti squash
- 1 cup marinara sauce (choose a low-sugar option)
- 2 cloves garlic, minced
- 1/4 cup chopped fresh basil leaves
- Salt and pepper to taste
- Grated Parmesan cheese for serving (optional)

Prep Time: 10 minutes
Cook Time: 40 minutes
Instructions:
- Preheat the oven to 400°F (200°C). Cut the spaghetti squash in half lengthwise and scoop out the seeds.
- Place the squash halves cut side down on a baking sheet lined with parchment paper.
- Bake in the preheated oven for 30-40 minutes, or until the squash is tender and easily pierced with a fork.
- While the squash is baking, heat the marinara sauce in a saucepan over medium heat. Stir in

the minced garlic and chopped basil. Simmer for 5 minutes.
- Scrape the cooked spaghetti squash strands with a fork and transfer to serving plates.
- Top with the tomato basil sauce.
- Serve hot, optionally garnished with grated Parmesan cheese.

Nutritional Values (per serving):
- Total Carbohydrate: 29g
- Dietary Fiber: 7g
- Total Sugars: 12g
- Protein: 4g
- Total Fat: 5g
- Saturated Fat: 1g
- Cholesterol: 0mg
- Vitamin A: 1128IU
- Vitamin C: 16mg
- Folate: 36mcg
- Sodium: 541mg
- Calcium: 71mg
- Iron: 2mg
- Magnesium: 72mg
- Potassium: 746mg

QUINOA-STUFFED BELL PEPPERS

Servings: 4
Ingredients:
- 4 large bell peppers, halved and seeded
- 1 cup cooked quinoa
- 1 cup black beans, drained and rinsed
- 1 cup corn kernels (fresh or frozen)
- 1/2 cup diced tomatoes
- 1/4 cup chopped fresh cilantro
- 1 teaspoon ground cumin
- 1/2 teaspoon chili powder
- Salt and pepper to taste
- 1/2 cup shredded cheddar cheese (optional)

Prep Time: 15 minutes
Cook Time: 30 minutes
Instructions:
- Preheat the oven to 375°F (190°C). Arrange the bell pepper halves in a baking dish.
- In a mixing bowl, combine the cooked quinoa, black beans, corn kernels, diced tomatoes, chopped cilantro, ground cumin, chili powder, salt, and pepper.

- Spoon the quinoa mixture evenly into each bell pepper half.
- Cover the baking dish with foil and bake in the preheated oven for 25-30 minutes, or until the peppers are tender.
- If using, sprinkle shredded cheddar cheese over the stuffed peppers during the last 5 minutes of baking.
- Serve hot.

Nutritional Values (per serving):
- Total Carbohydrate: 40g
- Dietary Fiber: 9g
- Total Sugars: 9g
- Protein: 11g
- Total Fat: 5g
- Saturated Fat: 2g
- Cholesterol: 9mg
- Vitamin A: 4542IU
- Vitamin C: 193mg
- Folate: 137mcg
- Sodium: 493mg
- Calcium: 162mg
- Iron: 3mg
- Magnesium: 99mg
- Potassium: 968mg

BROCCOLI AND MUSHROOM STIR-FRY

Servings: 4
Ingredients:
- 2 cups broccoli florets
- 2 cups sliced mushrooms
- 1 bell pepper, sliced
- 1 onion, sliced
- 2 cloves garlic, minced
- 2 tablespoons low-sodium soy sauce or tamari
- 1 tablespoon sesame oil
- 1 teaspoon cornstarch
- 1/4 cup water
- Sesame seeds for garnish (optional)

Prep Time: 10 minutes
Cook Time: 10 minutes
Instructions:
- In a small bowl, whisk together the low-sodium soy sauce, sesame oil, cornstarch, and water to make the sauce. Set aside.
- Heat a large skillet or wok over medium-high heat. Add a splash of oil if needed.

- Add the sliced mushrooms, bell pepper, and onion to the skillet. Stir-fry for 3-4 minutes until slightly softened.
- Add the minced garlic and broccoli florets to the skillet. Stir-fry for another 2-3 minutes.
- Pour the prepared sauce over the vegetables in the skillet. Stir well to coat.
- Cook for an additional 2-3 minutes until the sauce has thickened and the vegetables are tender-crisp.
- Garnish with sesame seeds if desired.
- Serve hot, optionally over cooked brown rice or quinoa.

Nutritional Values (per serving):
- Total Carbohydrate: 12g
- Dietary Fiber: 4g
- Total Sugars: 4g
- Protein: 5g
- Total Fat: 3g
- Saturated Fat: 0g
- Cholesterol: 0mg
- Vitamin A: 1276IU
- Vitamin C: 78mg
- Folate: 55mcg
- Sodium: 334mg
- Calcium: 40mg
- Iron: 1mg
- Magnesium: 31mg
- Potassium: 398mg

STUFFED PORTOBELLO MUSHROOMS WITH SPINACH AND RICOTTA

Servings: 2
Ingredients:

- 2 large portobello mushroom caps
- 1 cup fresh spinach leaves
- 1/2 cup ricotta cheese
- 1/4 cup grated Parmesan cheese
- 2 cloves garlic, minced
- 1/4 teaspoon red pepper flakes (optional)
- Salt and pepper to taste

Prep Time: 10 minutes
Cook Time: 20 minutes
Instructions:

- Preheat the oven to 375°F (190°C). Remove the stems from the portobello mushroom caps and gently scrape out the gills.
- In a skillet, wilt the spinach over medium heat for 2-3 minutes. Drain any excess liquid.
- In a mixing bowl, combine the wilted spinach, ricotta cheese, grated Parmesan cheese, minced garlic, red pepper flakes (if using), salt, and pepper.
- Spoon the spinach and ricotta mixture into each portobello mushroom cap.
- Place the stuffed mushrooms on a baking sheet lined with parchment paper.
- Bake in the preheated oven for 15-20 minutes, or until the mushrooms are tender and the filling is heated through.
- Serve hot.

Nutritional Values (per serving):

- Total Carbohydrate: 12g
- Dietary Fiber: 3g
- Total Sugars: 4g
- Protein: 16g
- Total Fat: 12g
- Saturated Fat: 7g
- Cholesterol: 40mg
- Vitamin A: 2209IU
- Vitamin C: 4mg
- Folate: 49mcg
- Sodium: 286mg
- Calcium: 357mg
- Iron: 2mg
- Magnesium: 39mg
- Potassium: 715mg

CHICKPEA AND VEGETABLE STIR-FRY

Servings: 4
Ingredients:

- 1 can (15 oz) chickpeas, drained and rinsed
- 2 cups mixed vegetables (such as bell peppers, broccoli, and snap peas), sliced
- 1 onion, sliced
- 2 cloves garlic, minced
- 2 tablespoons low-sodium soy sauce or tamari
- 1 tablespoon rice vinegar
- 1 teaspoon sesame oil
- 1/2 teaspoon cornstarch
- 1/4 cup water
- Sesame seeds for garnish (optional)

Prep Time: 10 minutes
Cook Time: 10 minutes
Instructions:

- In a small bowl, whisk together the low-sodium soy sauce, rice vinegar, sesame oil, cornstarch, and water to make the sauce. Set aside.
- Heat a large skillet or wok over medium-high heat. Add a splash of oil if needed.
- Add the sliced onion to the skillet and stir-fry for 2-3 minutes until softened.
- Add the mixed vegetables and minced garlic to the skillet. Stir-fry for another 3-4 minutes until the vegetables are tender-crisp.
- Add the drained chickpeas to the skillet and pour the prepared sauce over the mixture. Stir well to coat.
- Cook for an additional 2-3 minutes until the sauce has thickened slightly.
- Garnish with sesame seeds if desired.
- Serve hot, optionally over cooked brown rice or quinoa.

Nutritional Values (per serving):

- Total Carbohydrate: 27g
- Dietary Fiber: 7g
- Total Sugars: 5g
- Protein: 9g
- Total Fat: 4g
- Saturated Fat: 1g
- Cholesterol: 0mg
- Vitamin A: 3586IU
- Vitamin C: 28mg

- Folate: 81mcg
- Sodium: 372mg
- Calcium: 66mg
- Iron: 3mg
- Magnesium: 62mg
- Potassium: 392mg

MEDITERRANEAN CHICKPEA SALAD

Servings: 4
Ingredients:
- 2 cups cooked chickpeas
- 1 cucumber, diced
- 1 cup cherry tomatoes, halved
- 1/4 cup chopped red onion
- 1/4 cup chopped fresh parsley
- 2 tablespoons lemon juice
- 2 tablespoons extra virgin olive oil
- 1 teaspoon dried oregano
- Salt and pepper to taste
- Crumbled feta cheese for serving (optional)

Prep Time: 10 minutes
Cook Time: 0 minutes
Instructions:
- In a large mixing bowl, combine the cooked chickpeas, diced cucumber, cherry tomatoes, chopped red onion, and chopped fresh parsley.
- In a small bowl, whisk together the lemon juice, extra virgin olive oil, dried oregano, salt, and pepper to make the dressing.
- Pour the dressing over the chickpea salad and toss gently to coat.
- Taste and adjust seasoning as needed.
- Serve chilled or at room temperature, optionally garnished with crumbled feta cheese.

Nutritional Values (per serving):
- Total Carbohydrate: 22g
- Dietary Fiber: 7g
- Total Sugars: 5g
- Protein: 7g
- Total Fat: 9g
- Saturated Fat: 1g
- Cholesterol: 0mg
- Vitamin A: 816IU
- Vitamin C: 22mg
- Folate: 92mcg
- Sodium: 148mg

- Calcium: 62mg
- Iron: 2mg
- Magnesium: 45mg
- Potassium: 396mg

TOFU AND VEGETABLE STIR-FRY

Servings: 4
Ingredients:
- 1 block (14 oz) extra firm tofu, drained and cubed
- 2 cups mixed vegetables (such as bell peppers, broccoli, and snow peas), sliced
- 1 onion, sliced
- 2 cloves garlic, minced
- 2 tablespoons low-sodium soy sauce or tamari
- 1 tablespoon hoisin sauce
- 1 tablespoon rice vinegar
- 1 teaspoon sesame oil
- 1/2 teaspoon cornstarch
- 1/4 cup water
- Sesame seeds for garnish (optional)

Prep Time: 15 minutes
Cook Time: 15 minutes
Instructions:
- In a small bowl, whisk together the low-sodium soy sauce, hoisin sauce, rice vinegar, sesame oil, cornstarch, and water to make the sauce. Set aside.
- Heat a large skillet or wok over medium-high heat. Add a splash of oil if needed.
- Add the cubed tofu to the skillet and cook for 5-6 minutes, stirring occasionally, until lightly browned.
- Remove the tofu from the skillet and set aside.
- Add the sliced onion to the skillet and stir-fry for 2-3 minutes until softened.
- Add the mixed vegetables and minced garlic to the skillet. Stir-fry for another 3-4 minutes until the vegetables are tender-crisp.
- Return the cooked tofu to the skillet and pour the prepared sauce over the mixture. Stir well to coat.
- Cook for an additional 2-3 minutes until the sauce has thickened slightly.
- Garnish with sesame seeds if desired.
- Serve hot, optionally over cooked brown rice or quinoa.

Nutritional Values (per serving):

- Total Carbohydrate: 16g
- Dietary Fiber: 4g
- Total Sugars: 5g
- Protein: 15g
- Total Fat: 9g
- Saturated Fat: 1g
- Cholesterol: 0mg
- Vitamin A: 3524IU
- Vitamin C: 27mg
- Folate: 64mcg
- Sodium: 373mg
- Calcium: 204mg
- Iron: 3mg
- Magnesium: 81mg
- Potassium: 535mg

LENTIL AND SPINACH SOUP

Servings: 4
Ingredients:

- 1 cup dried green lentils, rinsed and drained
- 4 cups vegetable broth
- 2 cups chopped fresh spinach leaves
- 1 onion, diced
- 2 carrots, diced
- 2 stalks celery, diced
- 2 cloves garlic, minced
- 1 teaspoon ground cumin
- 1/2 teaspoon smoked paprika
- Salt and pepper to taste
- Fresh lemon juice for serving (optional)

Prep Time: 10 minutes
Cook Time: 30 minutes
Instructions:

- In a large pot, combine the dried green lentils and vegetable broth. Bring to a boil over medium-high heat.
- Reduce the heat to low, cover, and simmer for 15 minutes.
- Add the diced onion, carrots, celery, minced garlic, ground cumin, smoked paprika, salt, and pepper to the pot.
- Continue to simmer for another 15 minutes, or until the lentils and vegetables are tender.
- Stir in the chopped fresh spinach leaves and cook for an additional 2-3 minutes until wilted.
- Taste and adjust seasoning as needed.

- Serve hot, optionally with a squeeze of fresh lemon juice.

Nutritional Values (per serving):

- Total Carbohydrate: 32g
- Dietary Fiber: 14g
- Total Sugars: 4g
- Protein: 14g
- Total Fat: 1g
- Saturated Fat: 0g
- Cholesterol: 0mg
- Vitamin A: 5594IU
- Vitamin C: 11mg
- Folate: 358mcg
- Sodium: 962mg
- Calcium: 101mg
- Iron: 5mg
- Magnesium: 72mg
- Potassium: 857mg

CAULIFLOWER FRIED RICE

Servings: 4
Ingredients:

- 1 medium head cauliflower, grated or finely chopped
- 2 eggs, lightly beaten
- 1 cup mixed vegetables (such as peas, carrots, and bell peppers), diced
- 1 onion, diced
- 2 cloves garlic, minced
- 2 tablespoons low-sodium soy sauce or tamari
- 1 tablespoon sesame oil
- 1 teaspoon grated ginger
- 2 green onions, thinly sliced (for garnish)

Prep Time: 15 minutes
Cook Time: 15 minutes
Instructions:

- In a large skillet or wok, heat half of the sesame oil over medium heat. Add the beaten eggs and scramble until cooked through. Remove from the skillet and set aside.
- Heat the remaining sesame oil in the skillet. Add the diced onion and mixed vegetables. Stir-fry for 3-4 minutes until softened.
- Add the minced garlic and grated ginger to the skillet. Stir-fry for another minute until fragrant.

- Add the grated cauliflower to the skillet. Stir-fry for 5-6 minutes until the cauliflower is tender.
- Return the cooked eggs to the skillet. Pour the low-sodium soy sauce over the mixture and stir well to combine.
- Cook for an additional 2-3 minutes until heated through.
- Garnish with thinly sliced green onions.
- Serve hot.

Nutritional Values (per serving):
- Total Carbohydrate: 16g
- Dietary Fiber: 6g
- Total Sugars: 6g
- Protein: 9g
- Total Fat: 7g
- Saturated Fat: 1g
- Cholesterol: 93mg
- Vitamin A: 4306IU
- Vitamin C: 69mg
- Folate: 118mcg
- Sodium: 380mg
- Calcium: 71mg
- Iron: 2mg
- Magnesium: 41mg
- Potassium: 654mg

CHAPTER 4
FISH AND SEAFOOD

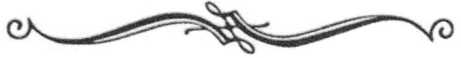

LEMON GARLIC BAKED SALMON

Servings: 2
Ingredients:
- 2 salmon fillets (6 oz each)
- 2 tablespoons olive oil
- 2 cloves garlic, minced
- 1 lemon, thinly sliced
- 1 tablespoon fresh lemon juice
- 1 teaspoon dried oregano
- Salt and pepper to taste
- Fresh parsley for garnish

Prep Time: 10 minutes
Cook Time: 15 minutes
Instructions:
- Preheat the oven to 375°F (190°C). Line a baking sheet with parchment paper.
- Place the salmon fillets on the prepared baking sheet. Drizzle with olive oil and sprinkle minced garlic over the top.
- Arrange lemon slices over the salmon fillets. Squeeze fresh lemon juice over each fillet.
- Sprinkle dried oregano, salt, and pepper evenly over the salmon.
- Bake in the preheated oven for 12-15 minutes, or until the salmon flakes easily with a fork.
- Garnish with fresh parsley before serving.

Nutritional Values (per serving):
- Total Carbohydrate: 3g
- Dietary Fiber: 1g
- Total Sugars: 0g
- Protein: 38g
- Total Fat: 20g
- Saturated Fat: 3g
- Cholesterol: 94mg
- Vitamin A: 139IU
- Vitamin C: 15mg
- Folate: 23mcg
- Sodium: 74mg
- Calcium: 32mg
- Iron: 1mg
- Magnesium: 62mg
- Potassium: 879mg

GARLIC BUTTER SHRIMP

Servings: 2
Ingredients:
- 1/2 lb large shrimp, peeled and deveined
- 2 tablespoons unsalted butter
- 2 cloves garlic, minced
- 1 tablespoon chopped fresh parsley
- 1 tablespoon lemon juice
- Salt and pepper to taste

Prep Time: 10 minutes
Cook Time: 5 minutes
Instructions:
- Heat the butter in a large skillet over medium-high heat. Add the minced garlic and sauté for 1 minute until fragrant.
- Add the shrimp to the skillet in a single layer. Cook for 2-3 minutes per side until pink and opaque.
- Stir in the chopped fresh parsley and lemon juice. Season with salt and pepper to taste.
- Cook for another minute, stirring occasionally.
- Remove from heat and transfer the shrimp to a serving plate.
- Serve hot, optionally garnished with additional chopped parsley and lemon wedges.

Nutritional Values (per serving):
- Total Carbohydrate: 2g
- Dietary Fiber: 0g
- Total Sugars: 0g
- Protein: 23g
- Total Fat: 9g
- Saturated Fat: 5g
- Cholesterol: 218mg
- Vitamin A: 446IU
- Vitamin C: 6mg

- Folate: 5mcg
- Sodium: 290mg
- Calcium: 41mg
- Iron: 2mg
- Magnesium: 31mg
- Potassium: 181mg

GRILLED LEMON HERB TILAPIA

Servings: 2
Ingredients:
- 2 tilapia fillets (6 oz each)
- 2 tablespoons olive oil
- 2 tablespoons fresh lemon juice
- 1 teaspoon dried thyme
- 1 teaspoon dried parsley
- 1/2 teaspoon garlic powder
- Salt and pepper to taste

Prep Time: 10 minutes
Cook Time: 8 minutes
Instructions:
- Preheat the grill to medium-high heat.
- In a small bowl, whisk together olive oil, lemon juice, dried thyme, dried parsley, garlic powder, salt, and pepper to make the marinade.
- Place the tilapia fillets in a shallow dish and pour the marinade over them. Turn to coat evenly.
- Let the fish marinate for 10 minutes.
- Remove the tilapia from the marinade and discard any excess marinade.
- Grill the tilapia fillets for 4 minutes per side, or until the fish flakes easily with a fork.
- Remove from the grill and serve hot.

Nutritional Values (per serving):
- Total Carbohydrate: 2g
- Dietary Fiber: 0g
- Total Sugars: 0g
- Protein: 24g
- Total Fat: 12g
- Saturated Fat: 2g
- Cholesterol: 57mg
- Vitamin A: 166IU
- Vitamin C: 4mg
- Folate: 6mcg
- Sodium: 66mg
- Calcium: 21mg
- Iron: 1mg

- Magnesium: 42mg
- Potassium: 406mg

BAKED LEMON GARLIC COD

Servings: 2
Ingredients:
- 2 cod fillets (6 oz each)
- 2 tablespoons olive oil
- 2 cloves garlic, minced
- 1 lemon, thinly sliced
- 1 tablespoon fresh lemon juice
- 1 teaspoon dried thyme
- Salt and pepper to taste
- Fresh parsley for garnish

Prep Time: 10 minutes
Cook Time: 15 minutes
Instructions:
- Preheat the oven to 375°F (190°C). Line a baking sheet with parchment paper.
- Place the cod fillets on the prepared baking sheet. Drizzle with olive oil and sprinkle minced garlic over the top.
- Arrange lemon slices over the cod fillets. Squeeze fresh lemon juice over each fillet.
- Sprinkle dried thyme, salt, and pepper evenly over the cod.
- Bake in the preheated oven for 12-15 minutes, or until the cod flakes easily with a fork.
- Garnish with fresh parsley before serving.

Nutritional Values (per serving):
- Total Carbohydrate: 3g
- Dietary Fiber: 1g
- Total Sugars: 0g
- Protein: 25g
- Total Fat: 14g
- Saturated Fat: 2g
- Cholesterol: 50mg
- Vitamin A: 159IU
- Vitamin C: 23mg
- Folate: 21mcg
- Sodium: 106mg
- Calcium: 43mg
- Iron: 1mg
- Magnesium: 37mg
- Potassium: 555mg

GARLIC PARMESAN BAKED SHRIMP

Servings: 2
Ingredients:

- 1/2 lb large shrimp, peeled and deveined
- 2 tablespoons unsalted butter, melted
- 2 cloves garlic, minced
- 1/4 cup grated Parmesan cheese
- 1 tablespoon chopped fresh parsley
- 1 tablespoon lemon juice
- Salt and pepper to taste

Prep Time: 10 minutes
Cook Time: 10 minutes
Instructions:

- Preheat the oven to 375°F (190°C). Line a baking sheet with parchment paper.
- In a mixing bowl, combine the melted butter, minced garlic, grated Parmesan cheese, chopped fresh parsley, lemon juice, salt, and pepper.
- Add the peeled and deveined shrimp to the bowl and toss to coat evenly.
- Arrange the shrimp in a single layer on the prepared baking sheet.
- Bake in the preheated oven for 8-10 minutes, or until the shrimp are pink and opaque.
- Serve hot, optionally garnished with additional chopped parsley and lemon wedges.

Nutritional Values (per serving):

- Total Carbohydrate: 1g
- Dietary Fiber: 0g
- Total Sugars: 0g
- Protein: 24g
- Total Fat: 10g
- Saturated Fat: 6g
- Cholesterol: 210mg
- Vitamin A: 429IU
- Vitamin C: 6mg
- Folate: 7mcg
- Sodium: 342mg
- Calcium: 182mg
- Iron: 2mg
- Magnesium: 47mg
- Potassium: 190mg

GRILLED TERIYAKI SALMON

Servings: 2
Ingredients:

- 2 salmon fillets (6 oz each)
- 1/4 cup low-sodium soy sauce or tamari
- 2 tablespoons honey or maple syrup
- 1 tablespoon rice vinegar
- 1 clove garlic, minced
- 1 teaspoon grated ginger
- Sesame seeds and sliced green onions for garnish

Prep Time: 10 minutes
Cook Time: 10 minutes
Instructions:

- In a small bowl, whisk together soy sauce, honey or maple syrup, rice vinegar, minced garlic, and grated ginger to make the teriyaki sauce.
- Place the salmon fillets in a shallow dish and pour half of the teriyaki sauce over them. Turn to coat evenly. Reserve the remaining sauce for later.
- Preheat the grill to medium-high heat. Grease the grill grates lightly to prevent sticking.
- Place the salmon fillets on the grill, skin-side down. Discard any excess marinade from the dish.
- Grill the salmon for 4-5 minutes per side, basting occasionally with the reserved teriyaki sauce, until cooked through.
- Transfer the grilled salmon to a serving plate.
- Garnish with sesame seeds and sliced green onions before serving.

Nutritional Values (per serving):

- Total Carbohydrate: 12g
- Dietary Fiber: 0g
- Total Sugars: 11g
- Protein: 36g
- Total Fat: 16g
- Saturated Fat: 3g
- Cholesterol: 94mg
- Vitamin A: 140IU
- Vitamin C: 1mg
- Folate: 5mcg
- Sodium: 914mg
- Calcium: 40mg
- Iron: 2mg
- Magnesium: 49mg
- Potassium: 649mg

LEMON HERB GRILLED SHRIMP SKEWERS

Servings: 4
Ingredients:
- 1 lb large shrimp, peeled and deveined
- 2 tablespoons olive oil
- 2 cloves garlic, minced
- Zest and juice of 1 lemon
- 1 tablespoon chopped fresh parsley
- 1 teaspoon dried oregano
- Salt and pepper to taste
- Wooden skewers, soaked in water for 30 minutes

Prep Time: 15 minutes
Cook Time: 6 minutes
Instructions:
- In a mixing bowl, combine olive oil, minced garlic, lemon zest and juice, chopped fresh parsley, dried oregano, salt, and pepper to make the marinade.
- Add the peeled and deveined shrimp to the bowl and toss to coat evenly.
- Thread the marinated shrimp onto the soaked wooden skewers, dividing evenly.
- Preheat the grill to medium-high heat. Grease the grill grates lightly to prevent sticking.
- Place the shrimp skewers on the grill and cook for 2-3 minutes per side, or until the shrimp are pink and opaque.
- Remove from the grill and serve hot.

Nutritional Values (per serving):
- Total Carbohydrate: 2g
- Dietary Fiber: 0g
- Total Sugars: 0g
- Protein: 24g
- Total Fat: 7g
- Saturated Fat: 1g
- Cholesterol: 190mg
- Vitamin A: 67IU
- Vitamin C: 5mg
- Folate: 6mcg
- Sodium: 233mg
- Calcium: 49mg
- Iron: 1mg
- Magnesium: 31mg
- Potassium: 219mg

BLACKENED CAJUN CATFISH

Servings: 2
Ingredients:
- 2 catfish fillets (6 oz each)
- 2 tablespoons Cajun seasoning
- 2 tablespoons olive oil
- Lemon wedges for serving

Prep Time: 5 minutes
Cook Time: 10 minutes
Instructions:
- Rub Cajun seasoning evenly over both sides of the catfish fillets.
- Heat olive oil in a large skillet over medium-high heat.
- Add the seasoned catfish fillets to the skillet and cook for 4-5 minutes per side, or until the fish flakes easily with a fork and is blackened on the outside.
- Serve hot, with lemon wedges on the side.

Nutritional Values (per serving):
- Total Carbohydrate: 0g
- Dietary Fiber: 0g
- Total Sugars: 0g
- Protein: 33g
- Total Fat: 17g
- Saturated Fat: 3g
- Cholesterol: 118mg
- Vitamin A: 1233IU
- Vitamin C: 0mg
- Folate: 10mcg
- Sodium: 102mg
- Calcium: 15mg
- Iron: 1mg
- Magnesium: 50mg
- Potassium: 526mg

OVEN-BAKED GARLIC PARMESAN TILAPIA

Servings: 2
Ingredients:

- 2 tilapia fillets (6 oz each)
- 2 tablespoons olive oil
- 2 cloves garlic, minced
- 1/4 cup grated Parmesan cheese
- 1 tablespoon chopped fresh parsley
- Salt and pepper to taste

Prep Time: 10 minutes
Cook Time: 15 minutes
Instructions:

- Preheat the oven to 400°F (200°C). Line a baking sheet with parchment paper.
- Place the tilapia fillets on the prepared baking sheet. Drizzle with olive oil and sprinkle minced garlic over the top.
- Sprinkle grated Parmesan cheese and chopped fresh parsley evenly over the tilapia fillets. Season with salt and pepper to taste.
- Bake in the preheated oven for 12-15 minutes, or until the fish flakes easily with a fork and the cheese is golden brown.
- Serve hot.

Nutritional Values (per serving):

- Total Carbohydrate: 1g
- Dietary Fiber: 0g
- Total Sugars: 0g
- Protein: 36g
- Total Fat: 16g
- Saturated Fat: 3g
- Cholesterol: 94mg
- Vitamin A: 140IU
- Vitamin C: 1mg
- Folate: 5mcg
- Sodium: 109mg
- Calcium: 44mg
- Iron: 2mg
- Magnesium: 48mg
- Potassium: 662mg

SHRIMP AND AVOCADO SALAD

Servings: 2
Ingredients:

- 1/2 lb cooked shrimp, peeled and deveined
- 1 avocado, diced
- 1 cup cherry tomatoes, halved
- 1/4 cup diced red onion
- 2 tablespoons chopped fresh cilantro
- 1 tablespoon olive oil
- 1 tablespoon lime juice
- Salt and pepper to taste

Prep Time: 10 minutes
Cook Time: 0 minutes
Instructions:

- In a large mixing bowl, combine the cooked shrimp, diced avocado, halved cherry tomatoes, diced red onion, and chopped fresh cilantro.
- In a small bowl, whisk together olive oil, lime juice, salt, and pepper to make the dressing.
- Pour the dressing over the shrimp and avocado mixture. Toss gently to coat.
- Taste and adjust seasoning as needed.
- Serve immediately.

Nutritional Values (per serving):

- Total Carbohydrate: 14g
- Dietary Fiber: 7g
- Total Sugars: 2g
- Protein: 27g
- Total Fat: 19g
- Saturated Fat: 3g
- Cholesterol: 214mg
- Vitamin A: 659IU
- Vitamin C: 26mg
- Folate: 96mcg
- Sodium: 381mg
- Calcium: 84mg
- Iron: 2mg
- Magnesium: 59mg
- Potassium: 900mg

BAKED DIJON MUSTARD SALMON

Servings: 2
Ingredients:
- 2 salmon fillets (6 oz each)
- 2 tablespoons Dijon mustard
- 1 tablespoon honey
- 1 tablespoon olive oil
- 1 tablespoon lemon juice
- Salt and pepper to taste

Prep Time: 10 minutes
Cook Time: 12 minutes
Instructions:
- Preheat the oven to 400°F (200°C). Line a baking sheet with parchment paper.
- In a small bowl, whisk together Dijon mustard, honey, olive oil, lemon juice, salt, and pepper to make the glaze.
- Place the salmon fillets on the prepared baking sheet. Brush the glaze over the top of each fillet.
- Bake in the preheated oven for 10-12 minutes, or until the salmon flakes easily with a fork.
- Serve hot.

Nutritional Values (per serving):
- Total Carbohydrate: 6g
- Dietary Fiber: 0g
- Total Sugars: 5g
- Protein: 36g
- Total Fat: 20g
- Saturated Fat: 3g
- Cholesterol: 94mg
- Vitamin A: 140IU
- Vitamin C: 2mg
- Folate: 6mcg
- Sodium: 159mg
- Calcium: 38mg
- Iron: 1mg
- Magnesium: 53mg
- Potassium: 774mg

MEDITERRANEAN GRILLED SWORDFISH

Servings: 2
Ingredients:
- 2 swordfish steaks (6 oz each)
- 2 tablespoons olive oil
- 1 lemon, juiced
- 2 cloves garlic, minced
- 1 teaspoon dried oregano
- Salt and pepper to taste

Prep Time: 10 minutes
Cook Time: 10 minutes
Instructions:
- In a small bowl, whisk together olive oil, lemon juice, minced garlic, dried oregano, salt, and pepper to make the marinade.
- Place the swordfish steaks in a shallow dish and pour the marinade over them. Turn to coat evenly.
- Let the fish marinate for 10-15 minutes.
- Preheat the grill to medium-high heat. Grease the grill grates lightly to prevent sticking.
- Place the swordfish steaks on the grill and cook for 4-5 minutes per side, or until the fish is cooked through and grill marks appear.
- Serve hot.

Nutritional Values (per serving):
- Total Carbohydrate: 2g
- Dietary Fiber: 0g
- Total Sugars: 0g
- Protein: 45g
- Total Fat: 21g
- Saturated Fat: 3g
- Cholesterol: 115mg
- Vitamin A: 138IU
- Vitamin C: 25mg
- Folate: 12mcg
- Sodium: 90mg
- Calcium: 35mg
- Iron: 1mg
- Magnesium: 94mg
- Potassium: 1018mg

COCONUT CURRY SHRIMP

Servings: 4
Ingredients:
- 1 lb large shrimp, peeled and deveined
- 1 tablespoon olive oil
- 1 onion, diced
- 2 cloves garlic, minced
- 1 red bell pepper, sliced
- 1 tablespoon curry powder
- 1 teaspoon ground turmeric
- 1 teaspoon ground cumin
- 1 can (14 oz) coconut milk
- Salt and pepper to taste
- Fresh cilantro for garnish

Prep Time: 10 minutes
Cook Time: 15 minutes
Instructions:
- Heat olive oil in a large skillet over medium heat. Add diced onion and minced garlic. Cook for 2-3 minutes until softened.
- Add sliced red bell pepper to the skillet and cook for another 2-3 minutes.
- Stir in curry powder, ground turmeric, and ground cumin. Cook for 1 minute until fragrant.
- Pour coconut milk into the skillet and bring to a simmer.
- Add peeled and deveined shrimp to the skillet. Cook for 5-6 minutes until the shrimp are pink and cooked through.
- Season with salt and pepper to taste.
- Garnish with fresh cilantro before serving.

Nutritional Values (per serving):
- Total Carbohydrate: 10g
- Dietary Fiber: 3g
- Total Sugars: 4g
- Protein: 26g
- Total Fat: 26g
- Saturated Fat: 19g
- Cholesterol: 191mg
- Vitamin A: 672IU
- Vitamin C: 40mg
- Folate: 32mcg
- Sodium: 224mg
- Calcium: 79mg
- Iron: 5mg
- Magnesium: 91mg
- Potassium: 684mg

HERB-CRUSTED BAKED HALIBUT

Servings: 2
Ingredients:
- 2 halibut fillets (6 oz each)
- 2 tablespoons olive oil
- 2 tablespoons chopped fresh parsley
- 1 tablespoon chopped fresh thyme
- 1 tablespoon grated Parmesan cheese
- 1 clove garlic, minced
- Salt and pepper to taste

Prep Time: 10 minutes
Cook Time: 15 minutes
Instructions:
- Preheat the oven to 400°F (200°C). Line a baking sheet with parchment paper.
- In a small bowl, combine olive oil, chopped fresh parsley, chopped fresh thyme, grated Parmesan cheese, minced garlic, salt, and pepper to make the herb crust.
- Place the halibut fillets on the prepared baking sheet. Brush the herb crust over the top of each fillet.
- Bake in the preheated oven for 12-15 minutes, or until the fish flakes easily with a fork and the crust is golden brown.
- Serve hot.

Nutritional Values (per serving):
- Total Carbohydrate: 0g
- Dietary Fiber: 0g
- Total Sugars: 0g
- Protein: 37g
- Total Fat: 20g
- Saturated Fat: 3g
- Cholesterol: 73mg
- Vitamin A: 376IU
- Vitamin C: 4mg
- Folate: 4mcg
- Sodium: 95mg
- Calcium: 63mg
- Iron: 1mg
- Magnesium: 83mg
- Potassium: 740mg

LEMON GARLIC BUTTER SCALLOPS

Servings: 2
Ingredients:
- 1/2 lb sea scallops
- 2 tablespoons unsalted butter
- 2 cloves garlic, minced
- Zest and juice of 1 lemon
- Salt and pepper to taste

Prep Time: 10 minutes
Cook Time: 5 minutes
Instructions:
- Pat the sea scallops dry with paper towels. Season both sides with salt and pepper.
- In a large skillet, melt the unsalted butter over medium-high heat. Add minced garlic and cook for 1 minute until fragrant.
- Add the sea scallops to the skillet in a single layer. Cook for 2-3 minutes per side until golden brown and cooked through.
- Remove the scallops from the skillet and transfer to a serving plate.
- Drizzle lemon juice over the scallops and sprinkle lemon zest on top.
- Serve hot.

Nutritional Values (per serving):
- Total Carbohydrate: 4g
- Dietary Fiber: 0g
- Total Sugars: 0g
- Protein: 23g
- Total Fat: 9g
- Saturated Fat: 5g
- Cholesterol: 68mg
- Vitamin A: 318IU
- Vitamin C: 4mg
- Folate: 3mcg
- Sodium: 591mg
- Calcium: 34mg
- Iron: 1mg
- Magnesium: 31mg
- Potassium: 356mg

CHAPTER 5
MEAT RECIPES

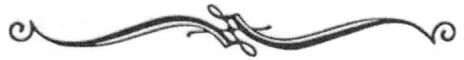

BALSAMIC GLAZED GRILLED CHICKEN BREAST

Servings: 2
Ingredients:
- 2 boneless, skinless chicken breasts (6 oz each)
- 2 tablespoons balsamic vinegar
- 1 tablespoon olive oil
- 2 cloves garlic, minced
- 1 teaspoon dried Italian herbs (such as oregano, basil, thyme)
- Salt and pepper to taste

Prep Time: 10 minutes
Cook Time: 12 minutes
Instructions:
- In a small bowl, whisk together balsamic vinegar, olive oil, minced garlic, dried Italian herbs, salt, and pepper to make the marinade.
- Place the chicken breasts in a shallow dish and pour the marinade over them. Turn to coat evenly.
- Let the chicken marinate for 30 minutes to 1 hour in the refrigerator.
- Preheat the grill to medium-high heat. Grease the grill grates lightly to prevent sticking.
- Remove the chicken breasts from the marinade and discard any excess marinade.
- Grill the chicken breasts for 6-7 minutes per side, or until cooked through and no longer pink in the center.
- Serve hot, optionally garnished with fresh herbs.

Nutritional Values (per serving):
- Total Carbohydrate: 3g
- Dietary Fiber: 0g
- Total Sugars: 2g
- Protein: 36g
- Total Fat: 9g
- Saturated Fat: 1g
- Cholesterol: 108mg
- Vitamin A: 26IU
- Vitamin C: 1mg
- Folate: 1mcg
- Sodium: 142mg
- Calcium: 20mg
- Iron: 1mg
- Magnesium: 38mg
- Potassium: 482mg

SLOW COOKER BEEF STEW

Servings: 4
Ingredients:
- 1 lb beef stew meat, cubed
- 4 cups low-sodium beef broth
- 2 potatoes, diced
- 2 carrots, sliced
- 1 onion, diced
- 2 cloves garlic, minced
- 1 teaspoon dried thyme
- Salt and pepper to taste

Prep Time: 15 minutes
Cook Time: 6 hours
Instructions:
- In a slow cooker, combine beef stew meat, low-sodium beef broth, diced potatoes, sliced carrots, diced onion, minced garlic, dried thyme, salt, and pepper.
- Cover and cook on low heat for 6 hours, or until the beef is tender and the vegetables are cooked through.
- Taste and adjust seasoning if needed before serving.
- Serve hot, optionally garnished with fresh parsley.

Nutritional Values (per serving):
- Total Carbohydrate: 21g
- Dietary Fiber: 3g

- Total Sugars: 4g
- Protein: 28g
- Total Fat: 10g
- Saturated Fat: 3g
- Cholesterol: 70mg
- Vitamin A: 5202IU
- Vitamin C: 14mg
- Folate: 30mcg
- Sodium: 267mg
- Calcium: 59mg
- Iron: 4mg
- Magnesium: 55mg
- Potassium: 919mg

- Total Sugars: 0g
- Protein: 29g
- Total Fat: 20g
- Saturated Fat: 6g
- Cholesterol: 92mg
- Vitamin A: 28IU
- Vitamin C: 10mg
- Folate: 6mcg
- Sodium: 62mg
- Calcium: 31mg
- Iron: 2mg
- Magnesium: 27mg
- Potassium: 399mg

LEMON GARLIC HERB GRILLED LAMB CHOPS

Servings: 2
Ingredients:
- 4 lamb loin chops (4 oz each)
- 2 tablespoons olive oil
- 2 cloves garlic, minced
- Zest and juice of 1 lemon
- 1 tablespoon chopped fresh rosemary
- Salt and pepper to taste

Prep Time: 10 minutes
Cook Time: 10 minutes
Instructions:
- In a small bowl, whisk together olive oil, minced garlic, lemon zest and juice, chopped fresh rosemary, salt, and pepper to make the marinade.
- Place the lamb loin chops in a shallow dish and pour the marinade over them. Turn to coat evenly.
- Let the lamb chops marinate for 30 minutes to 1 hour in the refrigerator.
- Preheat the grill to medium-high heat. Grease the grill grates lightly to prevent sticking.
- Remove the lamb chops from the marinade and discard any excess marinade.
- Grill the lamb chops for 4-5 minutes per side, or until cooked to your desired level of doneness.
- Serve hot, optionally garnished with additional chopped fresh rosemary.

Nutritional Values (per serving):
- Total Carbohydrate: 2g
- Dietary Fiber: 0g

TURKEY AND VEGETABLE STIR-FRY

Servings: 4
Ingredients:
- 1 lb turkey breast, thinly sliced
- 2 tablespoons low-sodium soy sauce or tamari
- 1 tablespoon hoisin sauce
- 1 tablespoon olive oil
- 2 cloves garlic, minced
- 1 onion, sliced
- 1 bell pepper, sliced
- 1 cup broccoli florets
- 1 cup snap peas
- Salt and pepper to taste

Prep Time: 15 minutes
Cook Time: 10 minutes
Instructions:
- In a small bowl, whisk together low-sodium soy sauce or tamari and hoisin sauce to make the sauce.
- Heat olive oil in a large skillet or wok over medium-high heat. Add minced garlic and cook for 1 minute until fragrant.
- Add thinly sliced turkey breast to the skillet and cook for 2-3 minutes until browned.
- Add sliced onion, sliced bell pepper, broccoli florets, and snap peas to the skillet. Cook for 3-4 minutes until the vegetables are tender-crisp.
- Pour the sauce over the turkey and vegetables in the skillet. Toss to coat evenly.
- Cook for an additional 1-2 minutes until heated through.
- Taste and adjust seasoning with salt and pepper if needed.

- Serve hot over cooked brown rice or quinoa if desired.

Nutritional Values (per serving):
- Total Carbohydrate: 10g
- Dietary Fiber: 3g
- Total Sugars: 4g
- Protein: 28g
- Total Fat: 7g
- Saturated Fat: 1g
- Cholesterol: 66mg
- Vitamin A: 1996IU
- Vitamin C: 78mg
- Folate: 58mcg
- Sodium: 494mg
- Calcium: 63mg
- Iron: 2mg
- Magnesium: 47mg
- Potassium: 595mg

HERB-ROASTED PORK TENDERLOIN

Servings: 4
Ingredients:
- 1 lb pork tenderloin
- 2 tablespoons olive oil
- 2 cloves garlic, minced
- 1 tablespoon chopped fresh rosemary
- 1 tablespoon chopped fresh thyme
- Salt and pepper to taste

Prep Time: 10 minutes
Cook Time: 25 minutes
Instructions:
- Preheat the oven to 400°F (200°C). Line a baking sheet with parchment paper.
- In a small bowl, combine olive oil, minced garlic, chopped fresh rosemary, chopped fresh thyme, salt, and pepper to make the herb mixture.
- Place the pork tenderloin on the prepared baking sheet. Rub the herb mixture over the entire surface of the pork.
- Roast in the preheated oven for 20-25 minutes, or until the internal temperature reaches 145°F (63°C) on a meat thermometer.
- Remove the pork tenderloin from the oven and let it rest for 5 minutes before slicing.
- Slice the pork tenderloin and serve hot.

Nutritional Values (per serving):
- Total Carbohydrate: 0g
- Dietary Fiber: 0g
- Total Sugars: 0g
- Protein: 36g
- Total Fat: 12g
- Saturated Fat: 3g
- Cholesterol: 111mg
- Vitamin A: 53IU
- Vitamin C: 1mg
- Folate: 1mcg
- Sodium: 67mg
- Calcium: 16mg
- Iron: 1mg
- Magnesium: 41mg
- Potassium: 618mg

TURKEY AND QUINOA STUFFED BELL PEPPERS

Servings: 4
Ingredients:
- 4 bell peppers, halved and seeds removed
- 1 lb ground turkey
- 1 cup cooked quinoa
- 1 onion, diced
- 2 cloves garlic, minced
- 1 can (14 oz) diced tomatoes, drained
- 1 teaspoon dried Italian herbs (such as oregano, basil, thyme)
- Salt and pepper to taste

Prep Time: 20 minutes
Cook Time: 40 minutes
Instructions:
- Preheat the oven to 375°F (190°C). Grease a baking dish with olive oil.
- In a large skillet, cook ground turkey over medium heat until browned. Drain any excess fat.
- Add diced onion and minced garlic to the skillet with the turkey. Cook for 2-3 minutes until softened.
- Stir in cooked quinoa, diced tomatoes, dried Italian herbs, salt, and pepper. Cook for an additional 2-3 minutes to combine flavors.
- Place bell pepper halves in the prepared baking dish. Spoon the turkey and quinoa mixture into each pepper half.

- Cover the baking dish with aluminum foil and bake in the preheated oven for 30-35 minutes, or until the peppers are tender.
- Remove foil and bake for an additional 5 minutes to brown the tops if desired.
- Serve hot.

Nutritional Values (per serving):
- Total Carbohydrate: 21g
- Dietary Fiber: 5g
- Total Sugars: 7g
- Protein: 30g
- Total Fat: 6g
- Saturated Fat: 1g
- Cholesterol: 62mg
- Vitamin A: 3479IU
- Vitamin C: 148mg
- Folate: 58mcg
- Sodium: 112mg
- Calcium: 60mg
- Iron: 3mg
- Magnesium: 65mg
- Potassium: 820mg

BEEF AND VEGETABLE KEBABS

Servings: 4
Ingredients:
- 1 lb beef sirloin, cut into 1-inch cubes
- 1 bell pepper, cut into chunks
- 1 onion, cut into chunks
- 1 zucchini, sliced
- 1/4 cup low-sodium soy sauce or tamari
- 2 tablespoons olive oil
- 2 cloves garlic, minced
- 1 teaspoon ground ginger
- Salt and pepper to taste

Prep Time: 20 minutes
Cook Time: 10 minutes
Instructions:
- In a shallow dish, combine low-sodium soy sauce or tamari, olive oil, minced garlic, ground ginger, salt, and pepper to make the marinade.
- Add beef sirloin cubes to the marinade and toss to coat. Cover and refrigerate for at least 30 minutes.
- Preheat the grill to medium-high heat. Thread marinated beef cubes, bell pepper chunks,

onion chunks, and zucchini slices onto skewers.
- Grill the kebabs for 8-10 minutes, turning occasionally, until the beef is cooked to your desired level of doneness and the vegetables are tender.
- Serve hot, optionally garnished with chopped fresh parsley.

Nutritional Values (per serving):
- Total Carbohydrate: 10g
- Dietary Fiber: 2g
- Total Sugars: 5g
- Protein: 32g
- Total Fat: 14g
- Saturated Fat: 4g
- Cholesterol: 94mg
- Vitamin A: 1088IU
- Vitamin C: 49mg
- Folate: 28mcg
- Sodium: 670mg
- Calcium: 38mg
- Iron: 4mg
- Magnesium: 57mg
- Potassium: 816mg

MOROCCAN SPICED CHICKEN THIGHS

Servings: 4
Ingredients:
- 4 chicken thighs, bone-in, skin-on
- 2 tablespoons olive oil
- 2 cloves garlic, minced
- 1 teaspoon ground cumin
- 1 teaspoon ground coriander
- 1/2 teaspoon ground cinnamon
- 1/4 teaspoon ground ginger
- 1/4 teaspoon ground paprika
- Salt and pepper to taste

Prep Time: 10 minutes
Cook Time: 25 minutes
Instructions:
- Preheat the oven to 400°F (200°C). Line a baking sheet with parchment paper.
- In a small bowl, combine olive oil, minced garlic, ground cumin, ground coriander, ground cinnamon, ground ginger, ground paprika, salt, and pepper to make the spice rub.

- Pat the chicken thighs dry with paper towels. Rub the spice rub all over the chicken thighs, ensuring they are evenly coated.
- Place the chicken thighs on the prepared baking sheet, skin side up.
- Bake in the preheated oven for 20-25 minutes, or until the chicken is cooked through and the skin is crispy.
- Serve hot, optionally garnished with chopped fresh cilantro.

Nutritional Values (per serving):
- Total Carbohydrate: 1g
- Dietary Fiber: 0g
- Total Sugars: 0g
- Protein: 23g
- Total Fat: 17g
- Saturated Fat: 4g
- Cholesterol: 110mg
- Vitamin A: 90IU
- Vitamin C: 1mg
- Folate: 3mcg
- Sodium: 72mg
- Calcium: 19mg
- Iron: 1mg
- Magnesium: 23mg
- Potassium: 268mg

TURKEY CHILI

Servings: 6
Ingredients:
- 1 lb ground turkey
- 1 onion, diced
- 2 cloves garlic, minced
- 1 bell pepper, diced
- 1 can (14 oz) diced tomatoes
- 1 can (15 oz) kidney beans, drained and rinsed
- 1 cup low-sodium chicken broth
- 2 tablespoons chili powder
- 1 teaspoon ground cumin
- Salt and pepper to taste

Prep Time: 15 minutes
Cook Time: 30 minutes
Instructions:
- In a large pot or Dutch oven, cook ground turkey over medium heat until browned.

- Add diced onion, minced garlic, and diced bell pepper to the pot with the turkey. Cook for 2-3 minutes until softened.
- Stir in diced tomatoes, kidney beans, low-sodium chicken broth, chili powder, ground cumin, salt, and pepper.
- Bring the chili to a simmer and let it cook for 20-25 minutes, stirring occasionally, until flavors are well combined and the chili has thickened.
- Taste and adjust seasoning with additional salt and pepper if needed.
- Serve hot, optionally garnished with shredded cheese and chopped fresh cilantro.

Nutritional Values (per serving):
- Total Carbohydrate: 13g
- Dietary Fiber: 5g
- Total Sugars: 4g
- Protein: 21g
- Total Fat: 7g
- Saturated Fat: 2g
- Cholesterol: 62mg
- Vitamin A: 908IU
- Vitamin C: 22mg
- Folate: 27mcg
- Sodium: 465mg
- Calcium: 49mg
- Iron: 2mg
- Magnesium: 38mg
- Potassium: 495mg

HERB-CRUSTED PORK CHOPS

Servings: 4
Ingredients:
- 4 bone-in pork chops (6 oz each)
- 2 tablespoons Dijon mustard
- 1 tablespoon olive oil
- 2 cloves garlic, minced
- 1 tablespoon chopped fresh thyme
- 1 tablespoon chopped fresh rosemary
- Salt and pepper to taste

Prep Time: 10 minutes
Cook Time: 15 minutes
Instructions:
- Preheat the oven to 400°F (200°C). Line a baking sheet with parchment paper.

- In a small bowl, combine Dijon mustard, olive oil, minced garlic, chopped fresh thyme, chopped fresh rosemary, salt, and pepper to make the herb crust.
- Pat the pork chops dry with paper towels. Spread the herb crust evenly over each pork chop.
- Place the pork chops on the prepared baking sheet.
- Bake in the preheated oven for 12-15 minutes, or until the pork is cooked through and the crust is golden brown.
- Serve hot.

Nutritional Values (per serving):
- Total Carbohydrate: 1g
- Dietary Fiber: 0g
- Total Sugars: 0g
- Protein: 36g
- Total Fat: 9g
- Saturated Fat: 3g
- Cholesterol: 108mg
- Vitamin A: 16IU
- Vitamin C: 2mg
- Folate: 3mcg
- Sodium: 140mg
- Calcium: 39mg
- Iron: 1mg
- Magnesium: 34mg
- Potassium: 599mg

HERB-MARINATED GRILLED PORK TENDERLOIN

Servings: 4
Ingredients:
- 1 lb pork tenderloin
- 2 tablespoons olive oil
- 2 cloves garlic, minced
- 1 tablespoon chopped fresh thyme
- 1 tablespoon chopped fresh rosemary
- Zest and juice of 1 lemon
- Salt and pepper to taste

Prep Time: 10 minutes
Cook Time: 15 minutes
Instructions:
- In a small bowl, combine olive oil, minced garlic, chopped fresh thyme, chopped fresh rosemary, lemon zest, lemon juice, salt, and pepper to make the marinade.
- Pat the pork tenderloin dry with paper towels. Place it in a shallow dish and pour the marinade over it, turning to coat evenly.
- Cover and refrigerate for at least 30 minutes to marinate.
- Preheat the grill to medium-high heat. Remove the pork tenderloin from the marinade and discard any excess marinade.
- Grill the pork tenderloin for 6-7 minutes per side, or until it reaches an internal temperature of 145°F (63°C) on a meat thermometer.
- Let the pork rest for 5 minutes before slicing. Serve hot.

Nutritional Values (per serving):
- Total Carbohydrate: 1g
- Dietary Fiber: 0g
- Total Sugars: 0g
- Protein: 26g
- Total Fat: 10g
- Saturated Fat: 2g
- Cholesterol: 74mg
- Vitamin A: 28IU
- Vitamin C: 6mg
- Folate: 7mcg
- Sodium: 56mg
- Calcium: 17mg
- Iron: 1mg
- Magnesium: 24mg
- Potassium: 461mg

MEDITERRANEAN TURKEY MEATBALLS

Servings: 4
Ingredients:
- 1 lb ground turkey
- 1/4 cup breadcrumbs (whole wheat or gluten-free)
- 1/4 cup grated Parmesan cheese
- 2 cloves garlic, minced
- 1 teaspoon dried oregano
- 1 teaspoon dried basil
- 1/2 teaspoon smoked paprika
- Salt and pepper to taste

Prep Time: 15 minutes
Cook Time: 20 minutes
Instructions:

- Preheat the oven to 400°F (200°C). Line a baking sheet with parchment paper.
- In a large bowl, combine ground turkey, breadcrumbs, grated Parmesan cheese, minced garlic, dried oregano, dried basil, smoked paprika, salt, and pepper. Mix until well combined.
- Shape the mixture into golf ball-sized meatballs and place them on the prepared baking sheet.
- Bake in the preheated oven for 18-20 minutes, or until the meatballs are cooked through and lightly browned.
- Serve hot, optionally garnished with chopped fresh parsley and marinara sauce for dipping.

Nutritional Values (per serving):
- Total Carbohydrate: 5g
- Dietary Fiber: 1g
- Total Sugars: 1g
- Protein: 26g
- Total Fat: 9g
- Saturated Fat: 3g
- Cholesterol: 80mg
- Vitamin A: 107IU
- Vitamin C: 1mg
- Folate: 10mcg
- Sodium: 236mg
- Calcium: 72mg
- Iron: 1mg
- Magnesium: 25mg
- Potassium: 313mg

GARLIC AND HERB ROAST BEEF

Servings: 4
Ingredients:
- 1 lb beef roast (such as sirloin or tenderloin)
- 2 tablespoons olive oil
- 4 cloves garlic, minced
- 1 tablespoon chopped fresh rosemary
- 1 tablespoon chopped fresh thyme
- Salt and pepper to taste

Prep Time: 10 minutes
Cook Time: 45 minutes
Instructions:
- Preheat the oven to 375°F (190°C). Line a baking dish with aluminum foil.
- In a small bowl, combine olive oil, minced garlic, chopped fresh rosemary, chopped fresh thyme, salt, and pepper to make the herb mixture.
- Rub the herb mixture evenly over the surface of the beef roast.
- Place the beef roast in the prepared baking dish.
- Roast in the preheated oven for 40-45 minutes, or until the internal temperature reaches your desired level of doneness.
- Remove the beef roast from the oven and let it rest for 10 minutes before slicing.
- Slice the beef roast and serve hot.

Nutritional Values (per serving):
- Total Carbohydrate: 0g
- Dietary Fiber: 0g
- Total Sugars: 0g
- Protein: 23g
- Total Fat: 15g
- Saturated Fat: 4g
- Cholesterol: 78mg
- Vitamin A: 20IU
- Vitamin C: 2mg
- Folate: 3mcg
- Sodium: 49mg
- Calcium: 20mg
- Iron: 2mg
- Magnesium: 19mg
- Potassium: 299mg

CHAPTER 6
VEGETABLE ON SIDES

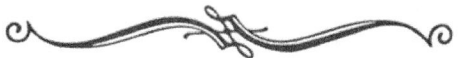

GARLIC ROASTED ASPARAGUS

Servings: 4
Ingredients:
- 1 lb asparagus spears, trimmed
- 2 tablespoons olive oil
- 4 cloves garlic, minced
- Salt and pepper to taste

Prep Time: 5 minutes
Cook Time: 15 minutes
Instructions:
- Preheat the oven to 400°F (200°C). Line a baking sheet with parchment paper.
- Place asparagus spears on the prepared baking sheet.
- Drizzle olive oil over the asparagus and sprinkle minced garlic on top. Toss to coat evenly.
- Season with salt and pepper to taste.
- Roast in the preheated oven for 12-15 minutes, or until the asparagus is tender and lightly browned.
- Serve hot.

Nutritional Values (per serving):
- Total Carbohydrate: 4g
- Dietary Fiber: 2g
- Total Sugars: 1g
- Protein: 2g
- Total Fat: 7g
- Saturated Fat: 1g
- Cholesterol: 0mg
- Vitamin A: 579IU
- Vitamin C: 7mg
- Folate: 68mcg
- Sodium: 75mg
- Calcium: 27mg
- Iron: 2mg
- Magnesium: 19mg
- Potassium: 229mg

LEMON GARLIC ROASTED BRUSSELS SPROUTS

Servings: 4
Ingredients:
- 1 lb Brussels sprouts, trimmed and halved
- 2 tablespoons olive oil
- Zest and juice of 1 lemon
- 4 cloves garlic, minced
- Salt and pepper to taste

Prep Time: 10 minutes
Cook Time: 25 minutes
Instructions:
- Preheat the oven to 400°F (200°C). Line a baking sheet with parchment paper.
- Place Brussels sprouts on the prepared baking sheet.
- In a small bowl, combine olive oil, lemon zest, lemon juice, minced garlic, salt, and pepper.
- Drizzle the olive oil mixture over the Brussels sprouts and toss to coat evenly.
- Arrange Brussels sprouts in a single layer on the baking sheet.
- Roast in the preheated oven for 20-25 minutes, or until the Brussels sprouts are tender and caramelized.
- Serve hot.

Nutritional Values (per serving):
- Total Carbohydrate: 8g
- Dietary Fiber: 3g
- Total Sugars: 2g
- Protein: 3g
- Total Fat: 7g
- Saturated Fat: 1g
- Cholesterol: 0mg
- Vitamin A: 600IU
- Vitamin C: 75mg
- Folate: 62mcg

- Sodium: 28mg
- Calcium: 38mg
- Iron: 1mg
- Magnesium: 23mg
- Potassium: 342mg

GARLIC PARMESAN ROASTED CAULIFLOWER

Servings: 4
Ingredients:
- 1 head cauliflower, cut into florets
- 2 tablespoons olive oil
- 4 cloves garlic, minced
- 1/4 cup grated Parmesan cheese
- Salt and pepper to taste

Prep Time: 10 minutes
Cook Time: 25 minutes
Instructions:
- Preheat the oven to 425°F (220°C). Line a baking sheet with parchment paper.
- Place cauliflower florets on the prepared baking sheet.
- In a small bowl, combine olive oil, minced garlic, grated Parmesan cheese, salt, and pepper.
- Drizzle the olive oil mixture over the cauliflower and toss to coat evenly.
- Spread cauliflower in a single layer on the baking sheet.
- Roast in the preheated oven for 20-25 minutes, or until the cauliflower is tender and golden brown.
- Serve hot.

Nutritional Values (per serving):
- Total Carbohydrate: 8g
- Dietary Fiber: 3g
- Total Sugars: 3g
- Protein: 4g
- Total Fat: 7g
- Saturated Fat: 2g
- Cholesterol: 4mg
- Vitamin A: 53IU
- Vitamin C: 69mg
- Folate: 64mcg
- Sodium: 138mg
- Calcium: 92mg
- Iron: 1mg
- Magnesium: 24mg

- Potassium: 472mg

ROASTED GARLIC MASHED CAULIFLOWER

Servings: 4
Ingredients:
- 1 head cauliflower, cut into florets
- 2 cloves garlic, peeled
- 2 tablespoons olive oil
- Salt and pepper to taste
- Chopped fresh chives for garnish (optional)

Prep Time: 10 minutes
Cook Time: 25 minutes
Instructions:
- Preheat the oven to 400°F (200°C). Line a baking sheet with parchment paper.
- Place cauliflower florets and whole garlic cloves on the prepared baking sheet.
- Drizzle olive oil over the cauliflower and garlic. Toss to coat evenly.
- Season with salt and pepper to taste.
- Roast in the preheated oven for 20-25 minutes, or until the cauliflower is tender and lightly browned.
- Transfer roasted cauliflower and garlic to a food processor. Pulse until smooth and creamy.
- Adjust seasoning if needed.
- Serve hot, garnished with chopped fresh chives if desired.

Nutritional Values (per serving):
- Total Carbohydrate: 6g
- Dietary Fiber: 3g
- Total Sugars: 2g
- Protein: 3g
- Total Fat: 7g
- Saturated Fat: 1g
- Cholesterol: 0mg
- Vitamin A: 3IU
- Vitamin C: 71mg
- Folate: 63mcg
- Sodium: 35mg
- Calcium: 32mg
- Iron: 1mg
- Magnesium: 23mg
- Potassium: 360mg

SAUTEED GARLIC GREEN BEANS

Servings: 4
Ingredients:
- 1 lb green beans, trimmed
- 2 tablespoons olive oil
- 4 cloves garlic, minced
- Salt and pepper to taste
- Balsamic Glazed Roasted Carrots

Prep Time: 5 minutes
Servings: 4
Ingredients:
- 1 lb carrots, peeled and sliced into sticks
- 2 tablespoons olive oil
- 2 tablespoons balsamic vinegar
- 1 tablespoon honey or maple syrup
- Salt and pepper to taste

Prep Time: 10 minutes
Cook Time: 25 minutes
Instructions:
- Preheat the oven to 400°F (200°C). Line a baking sheet with parchment paper.
- In a bowl, whisk together olive oil, balsamic vinegar, honey or maple syrup, salt, and pepper.
- Add the carrot sticks to the bowl and toss until evenly coated.
- Spread the carrots in a single layer on the prepared baking sheet.
- Roast in the preheated oven for 20-25 minutes, or until the carrots are tender and caramelized, stirring halfway through.
- Serve hot.

Nutritional Values (per serving):
- Total Carbohydrate: 13g
- Dietary Fiber: 3g
- Total Sugars: 7g
- Protein: 1g
- Total Fat: 7g
- Saturated Fat: 1g
- Cholesterol: 0mg
- Vitamin A: 19183IU
- Vitamin C: 7mg
- Folate: 22mcg
- Sodium: 81mg
- Calcium: 43mg
- Iron: 1mg

- Magnesium: 14mg
- Potassium: 361mg

GARLIC PARMESAN ROASTED BROCCOLI

Servings: 4
Ingredients:
- 1 lb broccoli florets
- 2 tablespoons olive oil
- 4 cloves garlic, minced
- 1/4 cup grated Parmesan cheese
- Salt and pepper to taste

Prep Time: 10 minutes
Cook Time: 20 minutes
Instructions:
- Preheat the oven to 425°F (220°C). Line a baking sheet with parchment paper.
- In a bowl, combine broccoli florets, olive oil, minced garlic, grated Parmesan cheese, salt, and pepper. Toss until evenly coated.
- Spread the broccoli in a single layer on the prepared baking sheet.
- Roast in the preheated oven for 18-20 minutes, or until the broccoli is tender and the edges are crispy.
- Serve hot.

Nutritional Values (per serving):
- Total Carbohydrate: 9g
- Dietary Fiber: 3g
- Total Sugars: 2g
- Protein: 4g
- Total Fat: 7g
- Saturated Fat: 2g
- Cholesterol: 4mg
- Vitamin A: 946IU
- Vitamin C: 101mg
- Folate: 63mcg
- Sodium: 149mg
- Calcium: 111mg
- Iron: 1mg
- Magnesium: 33mg
- Potassium: 431mg

LEMON GARLIC SAUTEED SPINACH

Servings: 4
Ingredients:

- 1 lb fresh spinach leaves
- 2 tablespoons olive oil
- 4 cloves garlic, minced
- Zest and juice of 1 lemon
- Salt and pepper to taste

Prep Time: 5 minutes
Cook Time: 5 minutes
Instructions:

- Heat olive oil in a large skillet over medium heat.
- Add minced garlic to the skillet and cook for 1 minute, or until fragrant.
- Add fresh spinach leaves to the skillet in batches, tossing until wilted.
- Once all the spinach is wilted, add lemon zest and lemon juice to the skillet. Toss to combine.
- Season with salt and pepper to taste.
- Cook for an additional 1-2 minutes, or until heated through.
- Serve hot.

Nutritional Values (per serving):

- Total Carbohydrate: 4g
- Dietary Fiber: 2g
- Total Sugars: 0g
- Protein: 3g
- Total Fat: 7g
- Saturated Fat: 1g
- Cholesterol: 0mg
- Vitamin A: 6228IU
- Vitamin C: 26mg
- Folate: 82mcg
- Sodium: 87mg
- Calcium: 95mg
- Iron: 3mg
- Magnesium: 79mg
- Potassium: 722mg

HONEY GLAZED ROASTED ROOT VEGETABLES

Servings: 4
Ingredients:

- 1 lb mixed root vegetables (carrots, parsnips, sweet potatoes), peeled and diced
- 2 tablespoons olive oil
- 2 tablespoons honey
- 1 teaspoon dried thyme
- Salt and pepper to taste

Prep Time: 10 minutes
Cook Time: 30 minutes
Instructions:

- Preheat the oven to 400°F (200°C). Line a baking sheet with parchment paper.
- In a bowl, combine diced root vegetables, olive oil, honey, dried thyme, salt, and pepper. Toss until evenly coated.
- Spread the root vegetables in a single layer on the prepared baking sheet.
- Roast in the preheated oven for 25-30 minutes, or until the vegetables are tender and caramelized, stirring halfway through.
- Serve hot.

Nutritional Values (per serving):

- Total Carbohydrate: 34g
- Dietary Fiber: 5g
- Total Sugars: 16g
- Protein: 2g
- Total Fat: 7g
- Saturated Fat: 1g
- Cholesterol: 0mg
- Vitamin A: 15884IU
- Vitamin C: 23mg
- Folate: 37mcg
- Sodium: 47mg
- Calcium: 60mg
- Iron: 1mg
- Magnesium: 30mg
- Potassium: 595mg

SESAME GARLIC STIR-FRIED GREEN BEANS

Servings: 4
Ingredients:
- 1 lb green beans, trimmed
- 2 tablespoons sesame oil
- 4 cloves garlic, minced
- 1 tablespoon soy sauce (low-sodium)
- 1 tablespoon sesame seeds
- Salt and pepper to taste

Prep Time: 10 minutes
Cook Time: 10 minutes
Instructions:
- Heat sesame oil in a large skillet or wok over medium-high heat.
- Add minced garlic to the skillet and cook for 1 minute, or until fragrant.
- Add green beans to the skillet and stir-fry for 5-7 minutes, or until tender-crisp.
- Stir in soy sauce and sesame seeds. Toss to coat evenly.
- Season with salt and pepper to taste.
- Cook for an additional 1-2 minutes, then remove from heat.
- Serve hot.

Nutritional Values (per serving):
- Total Carbohydrate: 8g
- Dietary Fiber: 3g
- Total Sugars: 2g
- Protein: 2g
- Total Fat: 7g
- Saturated Fat: 1g
- Cholesterol: 0mg
- Vitamin A: 705IU
- Vitamin C: 12mg
- Folate: 37mcg
- Sodium: 140mg
- Calcium: 60mg
- Iron: 1mg
- Magnesium: 24mg
- Potassium: 239mg

GRILLED LEMON GARLIC ZUCCHINI

Servings: 4
Ingredients:
- 2 large zucchini, sliced into rounds
- 2 tablespoons olive oil
- 2 cloves garlic, minced
- Zest and juice of 1 lemon
- Salt and pepper to taste

Prep Time: 10 minutes
Cook Time: 8 minutes
Instructions:
- Preheat the grill to medium-high heat.
- In a bowl, combine sliced zucchini, olive oil, minced garlic, lemon zest, lemon juice, salt, and pepper. Toss until evenly coated.
- Place the zucchini rounds on the grill grate.
- Grill for 3-4 minutes per side, or until tender and grill marks appear.
- Remove from the grill and transfer to a serving platter.
- Serve hot.

Nutritional Values (per serving):
- Total Carbohydrate: 5g
- Dietary Fiber: 2g
- Total Sugars: 3g
- Protein: 2g
- Total Fat: 7g
- Saturated Fat: 1g
- Cholesterol: 0mg
- Vitamin A: 262IU
- Vitamin C: 22mg
- Folate: 21mcg
- Sodium: 9mg
- Calcium: 26mg
- Iron: 1mg
- Magnesium: 28mg
- Potassium: 360mg

GARLIC HERB ROASTED BELL PEPPERS

Servings: 4
Ingredients:

- 2 bell peppers (red, yellow, or orange), sliced
- 2 tablespoons olive oil
- 4 cloves garlic, minced
- 1 tablespoon chopped fresh parsley
- 1 teaspoon dried thyme
- Salt and pepper to taste

Prep Time: 10 minutes
Cook Time: 20 minutes
Instructions:

- Preheat the oven to 400°F (200°C). Line a baking sheet with parchment paper.
- Place sliced bell peppers on the prepared baking sheet.
- In a bowl, combine olive oil, minced garlic, chopped fresh parsley, dried thyme, salt, and pepper. Toss until evenly coated.
- Spread the olive oil mixture over the bell peppers.
- Roast in the preheated oven for 15-20 minutes, or until the bell peppers are tender and slightly charred.
- Serve hot.

Nutritional Values (per serving):

- Total Carbohydrate: 8g
- Dietary Fiber: 3g
- Total Sugars: 4g
- Protein: 1g
- Total Fat: 7g
- Saturated Fat: 1g
- Cholesterol: 0mg
- Vitamin A: 2295IU
- Vitamin C: 160mg
- Folate: 25mcg
- Sodium: 6mg
- Calcium: 17mg
- Iron: 1mg
- Magnesium: 18mg
- Potassium: 296mg

HONEY GLAZED ROASTED BEETS

Servings: 4
Ingredients:

- 1 lb beets, peeled and diced
- 2 tablespoons olive oil
- 2 tablespoons honey
- 1 teaspoon dried thyme
- Salt and pepper to taste

Prep Time: 10 minutes
Cook Time: 35 minutes
Instructions:

- Preheat the oven to 400°F (200°C). Line a baking sheet with parchment paper.
- In a bowl, combine diced beets, olive oil, honey, dried thyme, salt, and pepper. Toss until evenly coated.
- Spread the beets in a single layer on the prepared baking sheet.
- Roast in the preheated oven for 30-35 minutes, or until the beets are tender and caramelized, stirring halfway through.
- Serve hot.

Nutritional Values (per serving):

- Total Carbohydrate: 22g
- Dietary Fiber: 3g
- Total Sugars: 18g
- Protein: 2g
- Total Fat: 7g
- Saturated Fat: 1g
- Cholesterol: 0mg
- Vitamin A: 45IU
- Vitamin C: 6mg
- Folate: 89mcg
- Sodium: 94mg
- Calcium: 20mg
- Iron: 1mg
- Magnesium: 39mg
- Potassium: 518mg

LEMON GARLIC SAUTEED SWISS CHARD

Servings: 4
Ingredients:
- 1 lb Swiss chard, stems removed and leaves chopped
- 2 tablespoons olive oil
- 4 cloves garlic, minced
- Zest and juice of 1 lemon
- Salt and pepper to taste

Prep Time: 10 minutes
Cook Time: 8 minutes
Instructions:
- Heat olive oil in a large skillet over medium heat.
- Add minced garlic to the skillet and cook for 1 minute, or until fragrant.
- Add Swiss chard leaves to the skillet and sauté for 5-7 minutes, or until wilted.
- Add lemon zest and lemon juice to the skillet. Toss to combine.
- Season with salt and pepper to taste.
- Cook for an additional 1-2 minutes, or until heated through.
- Serve hot.

Nutritional Values (per serving):
- Total Carbohydrate: 7g
- Dietary Fiber: 3g
- Total Sugars: 1g
- Protein: 2g
- Total Fat: 7g
- Saturated Fat: 1g
- Cholesterol: 0mg
- Vitamin A: 10686IU
- Vitamin C: 39mg
- Folate: 15mcg
- Sodium: 86mg
- Calcium: 102mg
- Iron: 2mg
- Magnesium: 81mg
- Potassium: 647mg

GARLIC HERB ROASTED MUSHROOMS

Servings: 4
Ingredients:
- 1 lb cremini mushrooms, cleaned and halved
- 2 tablespoons olive oil
- 4 cloves garlic, minced
- 1 tablespoon chopped fresh parsley
- 1 teaspoon dried thyme
- Salt and pepper to taste

Prep Time: 10 minutes
Cook Time: 20 minutes
Instructions:
- Preheat the oven to 400°F (200°C). Line a baking sheet with parchment paper.
- In a bowl, combine cremini mushrooms, olive oil, minced garlic, chopped fresh parsley, dried thyme, salt, and pepper. Toss until evenly coated.
- Spread the mushrooms in a single layer on the prepared baking sheet.
- Roast in the preheated oven for 15-20 minutes, or until the mushrooms are tender and golden brown.
- Serve hot.

Nutritional Values (per serving):
- Total Carbohydrate: 5g
- Dietary Fiber: 1g
- Total Sugars: 2g
- Protein: 3g
- Total Fat: 7g
- Saturated Fat: 1g
- Cholesterol: 0mg
- Vitamin A: 13IU
- Vitamin C: 3mg
- Folate: 15mcg
- Sodium: 7mg
- Calcium: 9mg
- Iron: 1mg
- Magnesium: 11mg
- Potassium: 425mg

HONEY GLAZED ROASTED TURNIPS

Servings: 4
Ingredients:
- 1 lb turnips, peeled and diced
- 2 tablespoons olive oil
- 2 tablespoons honey
- 1 teaspoon dried thyme
- Salt and pepper to taste

Prep Time: 10 minutes
Cook Time: 30 minutes
Instructions:
- Preheat the oven to 400°F (200°C). Line a baking sheet with parchment paper.
- In a bowl, combine diced turnips, olive oil, honey, dried thyme, salt, and pepper. Toss until evenly coated.
- Spread the turnips in a single layer on the prepared baking sheet.
- Roast in the preheated oven for 25-30 minutes, or until the turnips are tender and caramelized, stirring halfway through.
- Serve hot.

Nutritional Values (per serving):
- Total Carbohydrate: 17g
- Dietary Fiber: 3g
- Total Sugars: 11g
- Protein: 1g
- Total Fat: 7g
- Saturated Fat: 1g
- Cholesterol: 0mg
- Vitamin A: 16IU
- Vitamin C: 19mg
- Folate: 19mcg
- Sodium: 89mg
- Calcium: 50mg
- Iron: 1mg
- Magnesium: 20mg
- Potassium: 324mg

LEMON GARLIC ROASTED ARTICHOKES

Servings: 4
Ingredients:
- 2 large artichokes, trimmed and halved
- 2 tablespoons olive oil
- 4 cloves garlic, minced
- Zest and juice of 1 lemon
- Salt and pepper to taste

Prep Time: 15 minutes
Cook Time: 30 minutes
Instructions:
- Preheat the oven to 400°F (200°C). Line a baking sheet with parchment paper.
- Place artichoke halves on the prepared baking sheet.
- In a bowl, combine olive oil, minced garlic, lemon zest, lemon juice, salt, and pepper. Toss until evenly coated.
- Spoon the olive oil mixture over the artichokes, ensuring they are well coated.
- Roast in the preheated oven for 25-30 minutes, or until the artichokes are tender and lightly browned.
- Serve hot.

Nutritional Values (per serving):
- Total Carbohydrate: 12g
- Dietary Fiber: 5g
- Total Sugars: 1g
- Protein: 4g
- Total Fat: 7g
- Saturated Fat: 1g
- Cholesterol: 0mg
- Vitamin A: 80IU
- Vitamin C: 12mg
- Folate: 56mcg
- Sodium: 118mg
- Calcium: 60mg
- Iron: 2mg
- Magnesium: 56mg
- Potassium: 474mg

GINGER GARLIC STIR-FRIED BOK CHOY

Servings: 4
Ingredients:

- 1 lb baby bok choy, halved lengthwise
- 2 tablespoons olive oil
- 2 cloves garlic, minced
- 1 tablespoon minced fresh ginger
- 1 tablespoon soy sauce (low-sodium)
- Salt and pepper to taste

Prep Time: 10 minutes
Cook Time: 5 minutes
Instructions:

- Heat olive oil in a large skillet or wok over medium-high heat.
- Add minced garlic and ginger to the skillet and cook for 1 minute, or until fragrant.
- Add baby bok choy to the skillet and stir-fry for 3-4 minutes, or until tender-crisp.
- Stir in soy sauce. Toss to coat evenly.
- Season with salt and pepper to taste.
- Cook for an additional 1-2 minutes, then remove from heat.
- Serve hot.

Nutritional Values (per serving):

- Total Carbohydrate: 3g
- Dietary Fiber: 1g
- Total Sugars: 1g
- Protein: 1g
- Total Fat: 7g
- Saturated Fat: 1g
- Cholesterol: 0mg
- Vitamin A: 2887IU
- Vitamin C: 45mg
- Folate: 68mcg
- Sodium: 105mg
- Calcium: 144mg
- Iron: 1mg
- Magnesium: 19mg
- Potassium: 329mg

GARLIC ROASTED RADISHES

Servings: 4
Ingredients:

- 1 lb radishes, trimmed and halved
- 2 tablespoons olive oil
- 4 cloves garlic, minced
- Salt and pepper to taste

Prep Time: 10 minutes
Cook Time: 20 minutes
Instructions:

- Preheat the oven to 400°F (200°C). Line a baking sheet with parchment paper.
- Place radish halves on the prepared baking sheet.
- In a bowl, combine olive oil and minced garlic. Toss the radishes in the mixture until evenly coated.
- Spread the radishes in a single layer on the prepared baking sheet.
- Roast in the preheated oven for 15-20 minutes, or until the radishes are tender and lightly browned.
- Serve hot.

Nutritional Values (per serving):

- Total Carbohydrate: 3g
- Dietary Fiber: 1g
- Total Sugars: 1g
- Protein: 1g
- Total Fat: 7g
- Saturated Fat: 1g
- Cholesterol: 0mg
- Vitamin A: 5IU
- Vitamin C: 15mg
- Folate: 16mcg
- Sodium: 60mg
- Calcium: 24mg
- Iron: 1mg
- Magnesium: 8mg
- Potassium: 230mg

LEMON HERB GRILLED EGGPLANT

Servings: 4
Ingredients:

- 2 medium eggplants, sliced into rounds
- 2 tablespoons olive oil
- Zest and juice of 1 lemon
- 1 tablespoon chopped fresh parsley
- 1 teaspoon dried oregano
- Salt and pepper to taste

Prep Time: 10 minutes
Cook Time: 8 minutes
Instructions:

- Preheat the grill to medium-high heat.
- In a bowl, combine olive oil, lemon zest, lemon juice, chopped fresh parsley, dried oregano, salt, and pepper. Toss until evenly coated.
- Brush both sides of the eggplant rounds with the olive oil mixture.
- Place the eggplant rounds on the grill grate.
- Grill for 3-4 minutes per side, or until tender and grill marks appear.
- Remove from the grill and transfer to a serving platter.
- Serve hot.

Nutritional Values (per serving):

- Total Carbohydrate: 9g
- Dietary Fiber: 5g
- Total Sugars: 4g
- Protein: 2g
- Total Fat: 7g
- Saturated Fat: 1g
- Cholesterol: 0mg
- Vitamin A: 29IU
- Vitamin C: 6mg
- Folate: 22mcg
- Sodium: 7mg
- Calcium: 22mg
- Iron: 1mg
- Magnesium: 27mg
- Potassium: 302mg

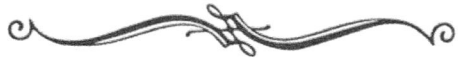

HEARTY VEGETABLE SOUP

Servings: 4
Ingredients:
- 1 tablespoon olive oil
- 1 onion, chopped
- 2 carrots, diced
- 2 celery stalks, diced
- 2 cloves garlic, minced
- 4 cups low-sodium vegetable broth
- 1 can (14 oz) diced tomatoes
- 1 can (15 oz) kidney beans, drained and rinsed
- 1 cup green beans, trimmed and chopped
- 1 teaspoon dried thyme
- Salt and pepper to taste

Prep Time: 10 minutes
Cook Time: 25 minutes
Instructions:
- Heat olive oil in a large pot over medium heat.
- Add chopped onion, diced carrots, and diced celery. Cook for 5-7 minutes, or until vegetables are softened.
- Add minced garlic and cook for 1 minute, or until fragrant.
- Pour in low-sodium vegetable broth and diced tomatoes. Bring to a simmer.
- Add kidney beans, chopped green beans, dried thyme, salt, and pepper. Stir to combine.
- Simmer for 15-20 minutes, or until vegetables are tender.
- Serve hot.

Nutritional Values (per serving):
- Total Carbohydrate: 30g
- Dietary Fiber: 9g
- Total Sugars: 7g
- Protein: 9g
- Total Fat: 4g
- Saturated Fat: 1g
- Cholesterol: 0mg

- Vitamin A: 6827IU
- Vitamin C: 22mg
- Folate: 74mcg
- Sodium: 658mg
- Calcium: 98mg
- Iron: 3mg
- Magnesium: 69mg
- Potassium: 654mg

CREAMY CAULIFLOWER SOUP

Servings: 4
Ingredients:
- 1 tablespoon olive oil
- 1 onion, chopped
- 2 cloves garlic, minced
- 1 head cauliflower, chopped
- 4 cups low-sodium vegetable broth
- 1/2 cup unsweetened almond milk
- Salt and pepper to taste

Prep Time: 10 minutes
Cook Time: 25 minutes
Instructions:
- Heat olive oil in a large pot over medium heat.
- Add chopped onion and cook for 5 minutes, or until softened.
- Add minced garlic and cook for 1 minute, or until fragrant.
- Add chopped cauliflower and low-sodium vegetable broth to the pot. Bring to a boil.
- Reduce heat and simmer for 15-20 minutes, or until cauliflower is tender.
- Use an immersion blender to puree the soup until smooth.
- Stir in unsweetened almond milk. Season with salt and pepper to taste.
- Simmer for an additional 5 minutes.
- Serve hot.

Nutritional Values (per serving):

- Total Carbohydrate: 11g
- Dietary Fiber: 4g
- Total Sugars: 4g
- Protein: 4g
- Total Fat: 4g
- Saturated Fat: 1g
- Cholesterol: 0mg
- Vitamin A: 143IU
- Vitamin C: 68mg
- Folate: 75mcg
- Sodium: 499mg
- Calcium: 99mg
- Iron: 1mg
- Magnesium: 28mg
- Potassium: 473mg

LENTIL SOUP

Servings: 4
Ingredients:
- 1 tablespoon olive oil
- 1 onion, chopped
- 2 carrots, diced
- 2 celery stalks, diced
- 2 cloves garlic, minced
- 1 cup dried green lentils, rinsed and drained
- 4 cups low-sodium vegetable broth
- 1 teaspoon ground cumin
- 1 teaspoon ground coriander
- Salt and pepper to taste

Prep Time: 10 minutes
Cook Time: 30 minutes
Instructions:
- Heat olive oil in a large pot over medium heat.
- Add chopped onion, diced carrots, and diced celery. Cook for 5-7 minutes, or until vegetables are softened.
- Add minced garlic, ground cumin, and ground coriander. Cook for 1 minute, or until fragrant.
- Add rinsed and drained green lentils and low-sodium vegetable broth to the pot. Bring to a boil.
- Reduce heat and simmer for 25-30 minutes, or until lentils are tender.
- Season with salt and pepper to taste.
- Serve hot.

Nutritional Values (per serving):
- Total Carbohydrate: 39g
- Dietary Fiber: 15g
- Total Sugars: 5g
- Protein: 15g
- Total Fat: 4g
- Saturated Fat: 1g
- Cholesterol: 0mg
- Vitamin A: 6905IU
- Vitamin C: 9mg
- Folate: 358mcg
- Sodium: 554mg
- Calcium: 68mg
- Iron: 5mg
- Magnesium: 96mg
- Potassium: 928mg

TOMATO BASIL SOUP

Servings: 4
Ingredients:
- 1 tablespoon olive oil
- 1 onion, chopped
- 2 cloves garlic, minced
- 2 cans (14 oz each) diced tomatoes
- 4 cups low-sodium vegetable broth
- 1/2 cup chopped fresh basil leaves
- Salt and pepper to taste

Prep Time: 10 minutes
Cook Time: 25 minutes
Instructions:
- Heat olive oil in a large pot over medium heat.
- Add chopped onion and cook for 5 minutes, or until softened.
- Add minced garlic and cook for 1 minute, or until fragrant.
- Add diced tomatoes (with juices) and low-sodium vegetable broth to the pot. Bring to a simmer.
- Simmer for 15-20 minutes, stirring occasionally.
- Use an immersion blender to puree the soup until smooth.
- Stir in chopped fresh basil leaves. Season with salt and pepper to taste.
- Simmer for an additional 5 minutes.
- Serve hot.

Nutritional Values (per serving):
- Total Carbohydrate: 14g
- Dietary Fiber: 3g
- Total Sugars: 8g
- Protein: 3g
- Total Fat: 4g
- Saturated Fat: 1g
- Cholesterol: 0mg
- Vitamin A: 1620IU
- Vitamin C: 23mg
- Folate: 29mcg
- Sodium: 536mg
- Calcium: 61mg
- Iron: 2mg
- Magnesium: 35mg
- Potassium: 676mg

BUTTERNUT SQUASH SOUP

Servings: 4
Ingredients:
- 1 tablespoon olive oil
- 1 onion, chopped
- 2 cloves garlic, minced
- 1 medium butternut squash, peeled, seeded, and chopped
- 4 cups low-sodium vegetable broth
- 1 teaspoon ground cinnamon
- 1/2 teaspoon ground nutmeg
- Salt and pepper to taste

Prep Time: 15 minutes
Cook Time: 30 minutes
Instructions:
- Heat olive oil in a large pot over medium heat.
- Add chopped onion and cook for 5 minutes, or until softened.
- Add minced garlic and cook for 1 minute, or until fragrant.
- Add chopped butternut squash and low-sodium vegetable broth to the pot. Bring to a boil.
- Reduce heat and simmer for 20-25 minutes, or until butternut squash is tender.
- Use an immersion blender to puree the soup until smooth.
- Stir in ground cinnamon and ground nutmeg. Season with salt and pepper to taste.
- Simmer for an additional 5 minutes.
- Serve hot.

Nutritional Values (per serving):
- Total Carbohydrate: 25g
- Dietary Fiber: 5g
- Total Sugars: 6g
- Protein: 2g
- Total Fat: 4g
- Saturated Fat: 1g
- Cholesterol: 0mg
- Vitamin A: 21418IU
- Vitamin C: 39mg
- Folate: 49mcg
- Sodium: 589mg
- Calcium: 116mg
- Iron: 1mg
- Magnesium: 48mg
- Potassium: 742mg

SPINACH AND WHITE BEAN SOUP

Servings: 4
Ingredients:
- 1 tablespoon olive oil
- 1 onion, chopped
- 2 cloves garlic, minced
- 4 cups low-sodium vegetable broth
- 1 can (15 oz) white beans, drained and rinsed
- 4 cups fresh spinach leaves
- 1 teaspoon dried oregano
- Salt and pepper to taste

Prep Time: 10 minutes
Cook Time: 20 minutes
Instructions:
- Heat olive oil in a large pot over medium heat.
- Add chopped onion and cook for 5 minutes, or until softened.
- Add minced garlic and cook for 1 minute, or until fragrant.
- Pour in low-sodium vegetable broth and bring to a simmer.
- Add drained and rinsed white beans to the pot. Simmer for 5 minutes.
- Stir in fresh spinach leaves and dried oregano. Cook until spinach wilts.
- Season with salt and pepper to taste.
- Serve hot.

Nutritional Values (per serving):
- Total Carbohydrate: 27g
- Dietary Fiber: 9g
- Total Sugars: 2g
- Protein: 10g
- Total Fat: 4g
- Saturated Fat: 1g
- Cholesterol: 0mg
- Vitamin A: 4333IU
- Vitamin C: 15mg
- Folate: 150mcg
- Sodium: 612mg
- Calcium: 157mg
- Iron: 4mg
- Magnesium: 102mg
- Potassium: 738mg

BROCCOLI CHEDDAR SOUP

Servings: 4
Ingredients:
- 1 tablespoon olive oil
- 1 onion, chopped
- 2 cloves garlic, minced
- 2 cups broccoli florets
- 4 cups low-sodium vegetable broth
- 1 cup unsweetened almond milk
- 1 cup shredded low-fat cheddar cheese
- Salt and pepper to taste

Prep Time: 10 minutes
Cook Time: 20 minutes
Instructions:
- Heat olive oil in a large pot over medium heat.
- Add chopped onion and cook for 5 minutes, or until softened.
- Add minced garlic and cook for 1 minute, or until fragrant.
- Add broccoli florets and low-sodium vegetable broth to the pot. Bring to a boil.
- Reduce heat and simmer for 10-15 minutes, or until broccoli is tender.
- Use an immersion blender to puree the soup until smooth.
- Stir in unsweetened almond milk and shredded low-fat cheddar cheese until cheese is melted.
- Season with salt and pepper to taste.
- Serve hot.

Nutritional Values (per serving):
- Total Carbohydrate: 12g
- Dietary Fiber: 3g
- Total Sugars: 4g
- Protein: 11g
- Total Fat: 9g
- Saturated Fat: 3g
- Cholesterol: 15mg
- Vitamin A: 1152IU
- Vitamin C: 60mg
- Folate: 62mcg
- Sodium: 499mg
- Calcium: 329mg
- Iron: 1mg
- Magnesium: 39mg
- Potassium: 522mg

SPICY BLACK BEAN SOUP

Servings: 4
Ingredients:
- 1 tablespoon olive oil
- 1 onion, chopped
- 2 cloves garlic, minced
- 2 cans (15 oz each) black beans, drained and rinsed
- 4 cups low-sodium vegetable broth
- 1 can (14 oz) diced tomatoes
- 1 teaspoon ground cumin
- 1/2 teaspoon chili powder
- Salt and pepper to taste

Prep Time: 10 minutes
Cook Time: 20 minutes
Instructions:
- Heat olive oil in a large pot over medium heat.
- Add chopped onion and cook for 5 minutes, or until softened.
- Add minced garlic and cook for 1 minute, or until fragrant.
- Add drained and rinsed black beans, low-sodium vegetable broth, diced tomatoes (with juices), ground cumin, and chili powder to the pot. Bring to a simmer.
- Simmer for 15-20 minutes, stirring occasionally.
- Use an immersion blender to puree a portion of the soup to desired consistency, leaving some beans whole.

- Season with salt and pepper to taste.
- Serve hot.

Nutritional Values (per serving):
- Total Carbohydrate: 30g
- Dietary Fiber: 12g
- Total Sugars: 4g
- Protein: 14g
- Total Fat: 4g
- Saturated Fat: 1g
- Cholesterol: 0mg
- Vitamin A: 645IU
- Vitamin C: 15mg
- Folate: 88mcg
- Sodium: 609mg
- Calcium: 111mg
- Iron: 4mg
- Magnesium: 95mg
- Potassium: 712mg

CREAMY MUSHROOM SOUP

Servings: 4
Ingredients:
- 1 tablespoon olive oil
- 1 onion, chopped
- 2 cloves garlic, minced
- 8 oz mushrooms, sliced
- 4 cups low-sodium vegetable broth
- 1/2 cup unsweetened almond milk
- 2 tablespoons nutritional yeast
- Salt and pepper to taste

Prep Time: 10 minutes
Cook Time: 25 minutes
Instructions:
- Heat olive oil in a large pot over medium heat.
- Add chopped onion and cook for 5 minutes, or until softened.
- Add minced garlic and sliced mushrooms. Cook for 8-10 minutes, or until mushrooms are tender and golden brown.
- Pour in low-sodium vegetable broth and bring to a simmer.
- Simmer for 10-15 minutes.
- Use an immersion blender to puree a portion of the soup to desired consistency, leaving some mushrooms whole.
- Stir in unsweetened almond milk and nutritional yeast until well combined.

- Season with salt and pepper to taste.
- Serve hot.

Nutritional Values (per serving):
- Total Carbohydrate: 11g
- Dietary Fiber: 3g
- Total Sugars: 3g
- Protein: 4g
- Total Fat: 5g
- Saturated Fat: 1g
- Cholesterol: 0mg
- Vitamin A: 186IU
- Vitamin C: 5mg
- Folate: 29mcg
- Sodium: 594mg
- Calcium: 66mg
- Iron: 1mg
- Magnesium: 19mg
- Potassium: 395mg

ROASTED RED PEPPER SOUP

Servings: 4
Ingredients:
- 1 tablespoon olive oil
- 1 onion, chopped
- 2 cloves garlic, minced
- 2 jars (12 oz each) roasted red peppers, drained
- 4 cups low-sodium vegetable broth
- 1/2 cup unsweetened almond milk
- Salt and pepper to taste

Prep Time: 10 minutes
Cook Time: 20 minutes
Instructions:
- Heat olive oil in a large pot over medium heat.
- Add chopped onion and cook for 5 minutes, or until softened.
- Add minced garlic and cook for 1 minute, or until fragrant.
- Add drained roasted red peppers and low-sodium vegetable broth to the pot. Bring to a simmer.
- Simmer for 10 minutes.
- Use an immersion blender to puree the soup until smooth.
- Stir in unsweetened almond milk until well combined.
- Season with salt and pepper to taste.
- Serve hot.

Nutritional Values (per serving):
- Total Carbohydrate: 12g
- Dietary Fiber: 2g
- Total Sugars: 5g
- Protein: 2g
- Total Fat: 4g
- Saturated Fat: 1g
- Cholesterol: 0mg
- Vitamin A: 98IU
- Vitamin C: 66mg
- Folate: 31mcg
- Sodium: 635mg
- Calcium: 76mg
- Iron: 1mg
- Magnesium: 17mg
- Potassium: 323mg

THAI COCONUT CURRY SOUP

Servings: 4
Ingredients:
- 1 tablespoon olive oil
- 1 onion, chopped
- 2 cloves garlic, minced
- 1 tablespoon grated ginger
- 2 tablespoons Thai red curry paste
- 4 cups low-sodium vegetable broth
- 1 can (14 oz) coconut milk
- 1 red bell pepper, sliced
- 1 cup sliced mushrooms
- 1 cup chopped kale
- 1 tablespoon soy sauce (or tamari for gluten-free)
- Juice of 1 lime
- Salt and pepper to taste

Prep Time: 10 minutes
Cook Time: 20 minutes
Instructions:
- Heat olive oil in a large pot over medium heat.
- Add chopped onion and cook for 5 minutes, or until softened.
- Add minced garlic, grated ginger, and Thai red curry paste. Cook for 1 minute, or until fragrant.
- Pour in low-sodium vegetable broth and coconut milk. Bring to a simmer.

- Add sliced red bell pepper, sliced mushrooms, and chopped kale to the pot. Simmer for 10-15 minutes, or until vegetables are tender.
- Stir in soy sauce and lime juice.
- Season with salt and pepper to taste.
- Serve hot.

Nutritional Values (per serving):
- Total Carbohydrate: 14g
- Dietary Fiber: 3g
- Total Sugars: 6g
- Protein: 4g
- Total Fat: 17g
- Saturated Fat: 13g
- Cholesterol: 0mg
- Vitamin A: 6994IU
- Vitamin C: 71mg
- Folate: 61mcg
- Sodium: 573mg
- Calcium: 77mg
- Iron: 3mg
- Magnesium: 55mg
- Potassium: 562mg

CREAMY ASPARAGUS SOUP

Servings: 4
Ingredients:
- 1 tablespoon olive oil
- 1 onion, chopped
- 2 cloves garlic, minced
- 1 lb asparagus, trimmed and chopped
- 4 cups low-sodium vegetable broth
- 1/2 cup unsweetened almond milk
- 2 tablespoons nutritional yeast
- Salt and pepper to taste

Prep Time: 10 minutes
Cook Time: 20 minutes
Instructions:
- Heat olive oil in a large pot over medium heat.
- Add chopped onion and cook for 5 minutes, or until softened.
- Add minced garlic and chopped asparagus. Cook for 5-7 minutes, or until asparagus is tender.
- Pour in low-sodium vegetable broth and bring to a simmer.
- Simmer for 10-15 minutes.

- Use an immersion blender to puree the soup until smooth.
- Stir in unsweetened almond milk and nutritional yeast until well combined.
- Season with salt and pepper to taste.
- Serve hot.

Nutritional Values (per serving):
- Total Carbohydrate: 11g
- Dietary Fiber: 4g
- Total Sugars: 4g
- Protein: 5g
- Total Fat: 5g
- Saturated Fat: 1g
- Cholesterol: 0mg
- Vitamin A: 1240IU
- Vitamin C: 11mg
- Folate: 86mcg
- Sodium: 607mg
- Calcium: 85mg
- Iron: 2mg
- Magnesium: 31mg
- Potassium: 428mg

ITALIAN WEDDING SOUP

Servings: 4
Ingredients:
- 1 tablespoon olive oil
- 1 onion, chopped
- 2 cloves garlic, minced
- 4 cups low-sodium chicken or vegetable broth
- 1/2 lb lean ground turkey or chicken
- 1/4 cup whole grain orzo pasta
- 2 cups chopped spinach leaves
- 1 egg, beaten
- 2 tablespoons grated Parmesan cheese
- Salt and pepper to taste

Prep Time: 10 minutes
Cook Time: 20 minutes
Instructions:
- Heat olive oil in a large pot over medium heat.
- Add chopped onion and cook for 5 minutes, or until softened.
- Add minced garlic and cook for 1 minute, or until fragrant.
- Pour in low-sodium chicken or vegetable broth and bring to a boil.

- Add lean ground turkey or chicken and whole grain orzo pasta to the pot. Cook for 8-10 minutes, or until meat is cooked through and pasta is tender.
- Stir in chopped spinach leaves and cook until wilted.
- Slowly pour beaten egg into the soup, stirring constantly to create egg ribbons.
- Stir in grated Parmesan cheese. Season with salt and pepper to taste.
- Serve hot.

Nutritional Values (per serving):
- Total Carbohydrate: 11g
- Dietary Fiber: 2g
- Total Sugars: 2g
- Protein: 21g
- Total Fat: 7g
- Saturated Fat: 2g
- Cholesterol: 95mg
- Vitamin A: 2468IU
- Vitamin C: 13mg
- Folate: 92mcg
- Sodium: 792mg
- Calcium: 126mg
- Iron: 3mg
- Magnesium: 44mg
- Potassium: 484mg

POTATO LEEK SOUP

Servings: 4
Ingredients:
- 1 tablespoon olive oil
- 2 leeks, white and light green parts only, sliced
- 2 cloves garlic, minced
- 2 large potatoes, peeled and diced
- 4 cups low-sodium vegetable broth
- 1/2 cup unsweetened almond milk
- Salt and pepper to taste

Prep Time: 10 minutes
Cook Time: 25 minutes
Instructions:
- Heat olive oil in a large pot over medium heat.
- Add sliced leeks and cook for 5 minutes, or until softened.
- Add minced garlic and cook for 1 minute, or until fragrant.

- Add diced potatoes and low-sodium vegetable broth to the pot. Bring to a boil.
- Reduce heat and simmer for 15-20 minutes, or until potatoes are tender.
- Use an immersion blender to puree the soup until smooth.
- Stir in unsweetened almond milk until well combined.
- Season with salt and pepper to taste.
- Serve hot.

Nutritional Values (per serving):
- Total Carbohydrate: 22g
- Dietary Fiber: 4g
- Total Sugars: 3g
- Protein: 3g
- Total Fat: 5g
- Saturated Fat: 1g
- Cholesterol: 0mg
- Vitamin A: 177IU
- Vitamin C: 26mg
- Folate: 39mcg
- Sodium: 622mg
- Calcium: 73mg
- Iron: 1mg
- Magnesium: 32mg
- Potassium: 592mg

LENTIL VEGETABLE SOUP

Servings: 4
Ingredients:
- 1 tablespoon olive oil
- 1 onion, chopped
- 2 cloves garlic, minced
- 1 carrot, diced
- 1 celery stalk, diced
- 1 cup dried green lentils, rinsed and drained
- 4 cups low-sodium vegetable broth
- 1 can (14 oz) diced tomatoes
- 1 teaspoon ground cumin
- 1 teaspoon dried thyme
- Salt and pepper to taste

Prep Time: 10 minutes
Cook Time: 30 minutes
Instructions:
- Heat olive oil in a large pot over medium heat.
- Add chopped onion and cook for 5 minutes, or until softened.

- Add minced garlic, diced carrot, and diced celery. Cook for 5 minutes, or until vegetables are tender.
- Add dried green lentils, low-sodium vegetable broth, diced tomatoes (with juices), ground cumin, and dried thyme to the pot. Bring to a boil.
- Reduce heat and simmer for 20-25 minutes, or until lentils are cooked through.
- Season with salt and pepper to taste.
- Serve hot.

Nutritional Values (per serving):
- Total Carbohydrate: 32g
- Dietary Fiber: 15g
- Total Sugars: 5g
- Protein: 16g
- Total Fat: 4g
- Saturated Fat: 1g
- Cholesterol: 0mg
- Vitamin A: 2558IU
- Vitamin C: 15mg
- Folate: 303mcg
- Sodium: 599mg
- Calcium: 76mg
- Iron: 5mg
- Magnesium: 80mg
- Potassium: 978mg

MINESTRONE SOUP

Servings: 4
Ingredients:
- 1 tablespoon olive oil
- 1 onion, chopped
- 2 cloves garlic, minced
- 1 carrot, diced
- 1 celery stalk, diced
- 1 zucchini, diced
- 1 can (14 oz) diced tomatoes
- 4 cups low-sodium vegetable broth
- 1/2 cup whole wheat pasta (small shapes like elbows or shells)
- 1 can (15 oz) cannellini beans, drained and rinsed
- 1 teaspoon dried basil
- 1 teaspoon dried oregano
- Salt and pepper to taste

Prep Time: 15 minutes
Cook Time: 25 minutes
Instructions:

- Heat olive oil in a large pot over medium heat.
- Add chopped onion and cook for 5 minutes, or until softened.
- Add minced garlic, diced carrot, diced celery, and diced zucchini. Cook for 5 minutes, or until vegetables are tender.
- Add diced tomatoes (with juices) and low-sodium vegetable broth to the pot. Bring to a boil.
- Add whole wheat pasta and cannellini beans to the pot. Cook for 10-12 minutes, or until pasta is al dente.
- Stir in dried basil and dried oregano. Season with salt and pepper to taste.
- Serve hot.

Nutritional Values (per serving):

- Total Carbohydrate: 49g
- Dietary Fiber: 12g
- Total Sugars: 7g
- Protein: 12g
- Total Fat: 4g
- Saturated Fat: 1g
- Cholesterol: 0mg
- Vitamin A: 5487IU
- Vitamin C: 30mg
- Folate: 175mcg
- Sodium: 532mg
- Calcium: 157mg
- Iron: 4mg
- Magnesium: 109mg
- Potassium: 972mg

CHAPTER 8
SALADS

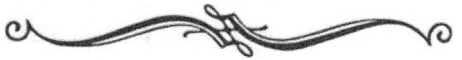

GRILLED CHICKEN CAESAR SALAD

Servings: 2
Ingredients:
- 2 boneless, skinless chicken breasts
- 1 tablespoon olive oil
- Salt and pepper to taste
- 1 head romaine lettuce, chopped
- 1/4 cup grated Parmesan cheese
- 1/2 cup whole wheat croutons
- Caesar dressing (store-bought or homemade)

Prep Time: 10 minutes
Cook Time: 15 minutes
Instructions:
- Preheat grill to medium-high heat.
- Brush chicken breasts with olive oil and season with salt and pepper.
- Grill chicken for 6-7 minutes per side, or until cooked through and no longer pink in the center.
- Remove chicken from grill and let rest for 5 minutes before slicing.
- In a large bowl, combine chopped romaine lettuce, grated Parmesan cheese, and whole wheat croutons.
- Add sliced grilled chicken on top of the salad.
- Drizzle with Caesar dressing and toss to coat evenly.
- Serve immediately.

Nutritional Values (per serving):
- Total Carbohydrate: 9g
- Dietary Fiber: 3g
- Total Sugars: 2g
- Protein: 29g
- Total Fat: 14g
- Saturated Fat: 4g
- Cholesterol: 82mg
- Vitamin A: 3724IU
- Vitamin C: 4mg
- Folate: 100mcg
- Sodium: 398mg
- Calcium: 205mg
- Iron: 2mg
- Magnesium: 37mg
- Potassium: 641mg

MEDITERRANEAN QUINOA SALAD

Servings: 4
Ingredients:
- 1 cup quinoa, rinsed
- 2 cups water or low-sodium vegetable broth
- 1 cucumber, diced
- 1 bell pepper, diced
- 1 cup cherry tomatoes, halved
- 1/4 cup sliced Kalamata olives
- 1/4 cup crumbled feta cheese
- 2 tablespoons chopped fresh parsley
- 2 tablespoons extra virgin olive oil
- Juice of 1 lemon
- Salt and pepper to taste

Prep Time: 10 minutes
Cook Time: 15 minutes
Instructions:
- In a medium saucepan, bring water or vegetable broth to a boil.
- Add rinsed quinoa, reduce heat to low, cover, and simmer for 12-15 minutes, or until quinoa is cooked and liquid is absorbed.
- Remove quinoa from heat and let cool for 5 minutes.
- In a large bowl, combine cooked quinoa, diced cucumber, diced bell pepper, halved cherry tomatoes, sliced Kalamata olives, crumbled feta cheese, and chopped fresh parsley.
- Drizzle extra virgin olive oil and lemon juice over the salad.
- Season with salt and pepper to taste.
- Toss to combine all ingredients evenly.
- Serve chilled or at room temperature.

Nutritional Values (per serving):
- Total Carbohydrate: 31g
- Dietary Fiber: 5g
- Total Sugars: 3g
- Protein: 8g
- Total Fat: 9g
- Saturated Fat: 2g
- Cholesterol: 6mg
- Vitamin A: 773IU
- Vitamin C: 38mg
- Folate: 92mcg
- Sodium: 259mg
- Calcium: 77mg
- Iron: 2mg
- Magnesium: 69mg
- Potassium: 378mg

GRILLED VEGETABLE SALAD

Servings: 4
Ingredients:
- 1 zucchini, sliced lengthwise
- 1 yellow squash, sliced lengthwise
- 1 red bell pepper, quartered
- 1 yellow bell pepper, quartered
- 1 red onion, sliced into rounds
- 1 tablespoon olive oil
- Salt and pepper to taste
- 4 cups mixed salad greens
- 1/4 cup crumbled goat cheese
- Balsamic vinaigrette (store-bought or homemade)

Prep Time: 10 minutes
Cook Time: 10 minutes
Instructions:
- Preheat grill to medium-high heat.
- Brush sliced zucchini, yellow squash, red bell pepper, yellow bell pepper, and red onion with olive oil. Season with salt and pepper.
- Grill vegetables for 3-4 minutes per side, or until grill marks appear and vegetables are tender.
- Remove vegetables from grill and let cool slightly.
- Chop grilled vegetables into bite-sized pieces.
- In a large bowl, combine mixed salad greens and chopped grilled vegetables.
- Sprinkle crumbled goat cheese over the salad.

- Drizzle with balsamic vinaigrette and toss to coat evenly.
- Serve immediately.

Nutritional Values (per serving):
- Total Carbohydrate: 9g
- Dietary Fiber: 3g
- Total Sugars: 5g
- Protein: 5g
- Total Fat: 7g
- Saturated Fat: 2g
- Cholesterol: 6mg
- Vitamin A: 1825IU
- Vitamin C: 105mg
- Folate: 49mcg
- Sodium: 141mg
- Calcium: 60mg
- Iron: 1mg
- Magnesium: 31mg
- Potassium: 366mg

STRAWBERRY SPINACH SALAD

Servings: 4
Ingredients:
- 4 cups baby spinach leaves
- 1 cup sliced strawberries
- 1/4 cup crumbled feta cheese
- 1/4 cup sliced almonds
- Balsamic vinaigrette (store-bought or homemade)

Prep Time: 10 minutes
Cook Time: 0 minutes
Instructions:
- In a large bowl, combine baby spinach leaves, sliced strawberries, crumbled feta cheese, and sliced almonds.
- Drizzle with balsamic vinaigrette and toss to coat evenly.
- Serve immediately.

Nutritional Values (per serving):
- Total Carbohydrate: 9g
- Dietary Fiber: 3g
- Total Sugars: 4g
- Protein: 5g
- Total Fat: 10g
- Saturated Fat: 2g
- Cholesterol: 11mg

- Vitamin A: 1815IU
- Vitamin C: 44mg
- Folate: 77mcg
- Sodium: 221mg
- Calcium: 138mg
- Iron: 2mg
- Magnesium: 68mg
- Potassium: 423mg

GREEK SALAD

Servings: 4
Ingredients:
- 4 cups chopped romaine lettuce
- 1 cucumber, diced
- 1 bell pepper, diced
- 1 cup cherry tomatoes, halved
- 1/4 cup sliced Kalamata olives
- 1/4 cup crumbled feta cheese
- 2 tablespoons chopped fresh parsley
- 2 tablespoons extra virgin olive oil
- 1 tablespoon red wine vinegar
- 1 teaspoon dried oregano
- Salt and pepper to taste

Prep Time: 10 minutes
Cook Time: 0 minutes
Instructions:
- In a large bowl, combine chopped romaine lettuce, diced cucumber, diced bell pepper, halved cherry tomatoes, sliced Kalamata olives, crumbled feta cheese, and chopped fresh parsley.
- In a small bowl, whisk together extra virgin olive oil, red wine vinegar, dried oregano, salt, and pepper.
- Drizzle dressing over the salad and toss to coat evenly.
- Serve immediately.

Nutritional Values (per serving):
- Total Carbohydrate: 9g
- Dietary Fiber: 3g
- Total Sugars: 4g
- Protein: 4g
- Total Fat: 10g
- Saturated Fat: 3g
- Cholesterol: 11mg
- Vitamin A: 2862IU

- Vitamin C: 47mg
- Folate: 78mcg
- Sodium: 346mg
- Calcium: 135mg
- Iron: 2mg
- Magnesium: 29mg
- Potassium: 377mg

CAPRESE SALAD

Servings: 4
Ingredients:
- 4 ripe tomatoes, sliced
- 8 oz fresh mozzarella cheese, sliced
- 1/4 cup fresh basil leaves
- 2 tablespoons extra virgin olive oil
- 1 tablespoon balsamic glaze
- Salt and pepper to taste

Prep Time: 10 minutes
Cook Time: 0 minutes
Instructions:
- On a serving platter, arrange alternating slices of tomatoes and fresh mozzarella cheese.
- Tuck fresh basil leaves between the tomato and mozzarella slices.
- Drizzle extra virgin olive oil and balsamic glaze over the salad.
- Season with salt and pepper to taste.
- Serve immediately.

Nutritional Values (per serving):
- Total Carbohydrate: 6g
- Dietary Fiber: 1g
- Total Sugars: 4g
- Protein: 8g
- Total Fat: 15g
- Saturated Fat: 7g
- Cholesterol: 34mg
- Vitamin A: 1162IU
- Vitamin C: 14mg
- Folate: 15mcg
- Sodium: 214mg
- Calcium: 190mg
- Iron: 1mg
- Magnesium: 22mg
- Potassium: 305mg

KALE AND QUINOA SALAD

Servings: 4
Ingredients:
- 1 cup quinoa, rinsed
- 2 cups water or low-sodium vegetable broth
- 4 cups chopped kale leaves
- 1/4 cup dried cranberries
- 1/4 cup chopped walnuts
- 1/4 cup crumbled feta cheese
- 2 tablespoons extra virgin olive oil
- 2 tablespoons balsamic vinegar
- Salt and pepper to taste

Prep Time: 10 minutes
Cook Time: 15 minutes
Instructions:
- In a medium saucepan, bring water or vegetable broth to a boil.
- Add rinsed quinoa, reduce heat to low, cover, and simmer for 12-15 minutes, or until quinoa is cooked and liquid is absorbed.
- Remove quinoa from heat and let cool for 5 minutes.
- In a large bowl, combine cooked quinoa, chopped kale leaves, dried cranberries, chopped walnuts, and crumbled feta cheese.
- Drizzle extra virgin olive oil and balsamic vinegar over the salad.
- Season with salt and pepper to taste.
- Toss to combine all ingredients evenly.
- Serve chilled or at room temperature.

Nutritional Values (per serving):
- Total Carbohydrate: 37g
- Dietary Fiber: 5g
- Total Sugars: 5g
- Protein: 9g
- Total Fat: 12g

- Saturated Fat: 2g
- Cholesterol: 6mg
- Vitamin A: 3645IU
- Vitamin C: 45mg
- Folate: 144mcg
- Sodium: 153mg
- Calcium: 152mg
- Iron: 3mg
- Magnesium: 105mg
- Potassium: 536mg

COBB SALAD

Servings: 4
Ingredients:
- 4 cups mixed salad greens
- 2 hard-boiled eggs, sliced
- 1 avocado, diced
- 1/2 cup cooked and diced chicken breast
- 1/4 cup crumbled blue cheese
- 1/4 cup diced tomatoes
- 1/4 cup diced cucumber
- 2 slices cooked turkey bacon, crumbled
- Balsamic vinaigrette (store-bought or homemade)

Prep Time: 15 minutes
Cook Time: 0 minutes
Instructions:
- In a large bowl, arrange mixed salad greens.
- Arrange sliced hard-boiled eggs, diced avocado, diced chicken breast, crumbled blue cheese, diced tomatoes, diced cucumber, and crumbled turkey bacon over the salad greens.
- Drizzle with balsamic vinaigrette.
- Serve immediately.

Nutritional Values (per serving):
- Total Carbohydrate: 9g
- Dietary Fiber: 4g
- Total Sugars: 2g
- Protein: 16g
- Total Fat: 27g
- Saturated Fat: 6g
- Cholesterol: 159mg
- Vitamin A: 2143IU
- Vitamin C: 11mg
- Folate: 85mcg
- Sodium: 265mg
- Calcium: 102mg
- Iron: 2mg
- Magnesium: 45mg
- Potassium: 676mg

TUNA SALAD

Servings: 4
Ingredients:

- 2 cans (5 oz each) tuna, drained
- 1/4 cup diced red onion
- 1/4 cup diced celery
- 1/4 cup diced red bell pepper
- 1/4 cup diced cucumber
- 1/4 cup diced dill pickles
- 1/4 cup plain Greek yogurt
- 1 tablespoon Dijon mustard
- 1 tablespoon lemon juice
- Salt and pepper to taste

Prep Time: 10 minutes
Cook Time: 0 minutes
Instructions:

- In a large bowl, combine drained tuna, diced red onion, diced celery, diced red bell pepper, diced cucumber, and diced dill pickles.
- In a small bowl, whisk together plain Greek yogurt, Dijon mustard, lemon juice, salt, and pepper.
- Pour the dressing over the tuna mixture and toss to coat evenly.
- Serve chilled or at room temperature.

Nutritional Values (per serving):

- Total Carbohydrate: 4g
- Dietary Fiber: 1g
- Total Sugars: 2g
- Protein: 21g
- Total Fat: 3g
- Saturated Fat: 1g
- Cholesterol: 42mg
- Vitamin A: 137IU
- Vitamin C: 17mg
- Folate: 7mcg
- Sodium: 338mg
- Calcium: 49mg
- Iron: 1mg
- Magnesium: 24mg
- Potassium: 236mg

ASIAN-INSPIRED EDAMAME SALAD

Servings: 4
Ingredients:

- 2 cups shelled edamame, cooked and cooled
- 1 red bell pepper, diced
- 1/2 cup shredded carrots
- 1/4 cup sliced scallions
- 1/4 cup chopped cilantro
- 2 tablespoons sesame seeds
- 2 tablespoons rice vinegar
- 1 tablespoon soy sauce (low-sodium)
- 1 tablespoon honey
- 1 tablespoon sesame oil
- 1 teaspoon grated ginger
- 1 clove garlic, minced

Prep Time: 10 minutes
Cook Time: 0 minutes
Instructions:

- In a large bowl, combine cooked and cooled shelled edamame, diced red bell pepper, shredded carrots, sliced scallions, chopped cilantro, and sesame seeds.
- In a small bowl, whisk together rice vinegar, soy sauce, honey, sesame oil, grated ginger, and minced garlic.
- Pour the dressing over the salad ingredients and toss to coat evenly.
- Serve chilled or at room temperature.

Nutritional Values (per serving):

- Total Carbohydrate: 13g
- Dietary Fiber: 5g
- Total Sugars: 5g
- Protein: 9g
- Total Fat: 7g
- Saturated Fat: 1g
- Cholesterol: 0mg
- Vitamin A: 2786IU
- Vitamin C: 58mg
- Folate: 106mcg
- Sodium: 245mg
- Calcium: 76mg
- Iron: 2mg
- Magnesium: 68mg
- Potassium: 407mg

CHAPTER 9
DESSERTS

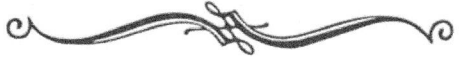

BERRY PARFAIT

Servings: 2
Ingredients:
- 1 cup mixed berries (such as strawberries, blueberries, raspberries)
- 1 cup low-fat Greek yogurt
- 2 tablespoons honey
- 1/4 cup granola (sugar-free)

Prep Time: 5 minutes
Cook Time: 0 minutes
Instructions:
- In serving glasses or bowls, layer mixed berries, low-fat Greek yogurt, and honey.
- Repeat the layers until all ingredients are used, finishing with a layer of berries on top.
- Sprinkle granola over the top layer.
- Serve immediately or refrigerate until ready to serve.

Nutritional Values (per serving):
- Total Carbohydrate: 33g
- Dietary Fiber: 4g
- Total Sugars: 25g
- Protein: 16g
- Total Fat: 2g
- Saturated Fat: 0g
- Cholesterol: 10mg
- Vitamin A: 157IU
- Vitamin C: 15mg
- Folate: 18mcg
- Sodium: 51mg
- Calcium: 185mg
- Iron: 1mg
- Magnesium: 26mg
- Potassium: 359mg

CHOCOLATE AVOCADO MOUSSE

Servings: 4
Ingredients:
- 2 ripe avocados
- 1/4 cup unsweetened cocoa powder
- 1/4 cup honey
- 1 teaspoon vanilla extract
- Pinch of salt

Prep Time: 10 minutes
Cook Time: 0 minutes
Instructions:
- Scoop the flesh of the avocados into a food processor.
- Add unsweetened cocoa powder, honey, vanilla extract, and a pinch of salt.
- Blend until smooth and creamy, scraping down the sides of the food processor as needed.
- Divide the mousse into serving dishes.
- Refrigerate for at least 30 minutes before serving.

Nutritional Values (per serving):
- Total Carbohydrate: 20g
- Dietary Fiber: 7g
- Total Sugars: 11g
- Protein: 3g
- Total Fat: 12g
- Saturated Fat: 2g
- Cholesterol: 0mg
- Vitamin A: 62IU
- Vitamin C: 6mg
- Folate: 52mcg
- Sodium: 4mg
- Calcium: 16mg
- Iron: 1mg
- Magnesium: 47mg
- Potassium: 487mg

APPLE CRISP

Servings: 6
Ingredients:
- 4 cups sliced apples (such as Granny Smith or Honeycrisp)
- 1 tablespoon lemon juice
- 1/2 teaspoon ground cinnamon
- 1/4 teaspoon ground nutmeg
- 1/4 cup old-fashioned oats
- 1/4 cup almond flour
- 1/4 cup chopped pecans
- 2 tablespoons honey
- 2 tablespoons melted coconut oil

Prep Time: 15 minutes
Cook Time: 30 minutes
Instructions:
- Preheat the oven to 350°F (175°C). Lightly grease a baking dish.
- In a large bowl, toss sliced apples with lemon juice, ground cinnamon, and ground nutmeg.
- Spread the apple mixture evenly in the prepared baking dish.
- In a separate bowl, combine old-fashioned oats, almond flour, chopped pecans, honey, and melted coconut oil.
- Sprinkle the oat mixture over the apples in the baking dish.
- Bake for 25-30 minutes, or until the topping is golden brown and the apples are tender.
- Serve warm.

Nutritional Values (per serving):
- Total Carbohydrate: 22g
- Dietary Fiber: 4g
- Total Sugars: 14g
- Protein: 2g
- Total Fat: 7g
- Saturated Fat: 3g
- Cholesterol: 0mg
- Vitamin A: 53IU
- Vitamin C: 5mg
- Folate: 7mcg
- Sodium: 1mg
- Calcium: 19mg
- Iron: 1mg
- Magnesium: 20mg
- Potassium: 174mg

CHIA SEED PUDDING

Servings: 4
Ingredients:
- 1/2 cup chia seeds
- 2 cups unsweetened almond milk
- 2 tablespoons honey or maple syrup
- 1 teaspoon vanilla extract
- Fresh berries for topping (optional)

Prep Time: 5 minutes
Cook Time: 0 minutes
Instructions:
- In a mixing bowl, whisk together chia seeds, unsweetened almond milk, honey or maple syrup, and vanilla extract.
- Let the mixture sit for 5 minutes, then whisk again to prevent clumps.
- Cover the bowl and refrigerate for at least 2 hours, or overnight, until the chia pudding thickens.
- Stir the pudding before serving and divide into serving cups.
- Top with fresh berries if desired.
- Serve chilled.

Nutritional Values (per serving):
- Total Carbohydrate: 13g
- Dietary Fiber: 9g
- Total Sugars: 6g
- Protein: 5g
- Total Fat: 8g
- Saturated Fat: 1g
- Cholesterol: 0mg
- Vitamin A: 43IU
- Vitamin C: 0mg
- Folate: 13mcg
- Sodium: 82mg
- Calcium: 332mg
- Iron: 2mg
- Magnesium: 91mg
- Potassium: 138mg

BANANA "ICE CREAM"

Servings: 2
Ingredients:
- 2 ripe bananas, sliced and frozen
- 2 tablespoons unsweetened almond milk
- 1 tablespoon cocoa powder (optional)
- Toppings of your choice (such as chopped nuts, shredded coconut, or dark chocolate chips)

Prep Time: 5 minutes
Cook Time: 0 minutes
Instructions:
- Place frozen banana slices in a blender or food processor.
- Add unsweetened almond milk and cocoa powder (if using).
- Blend until smooth and creamy, scraping down the sides as needed.
- Transfer the banana mixture to a bowl and fold in your favorite toppings.
- Serve immediately for a soft-serve consistency or freeze for 30 minutes for a firmer texture.

Nutritional Values (per serving):
- Total Carbohydrate: 27g
- Dietary Fiber: 3g
- Total Sugars: 14g
- Protein: 1g
- Total Fat: 1g
- Saturated Fat: 0g
- Cholesterol: 0mg
- Vitamin A: 76IU
- Vitamin C: 10mg
- Folate: 7mcg
- Sodium: 6mg
- Calcium: 10mg
- Iron: 0mg
- Magnesium: 27mg
- Potassium: 422mg

BAKED APPLES WITH CINNAMON

Servings: 4
Ingredients:
- 4 large apples (such as Gala or Fuji), cored
- 1 tablespoon honey or maple syrup
- 1 teaspoon ground cinnamon
- 1/4 cup chopped nuts (such as walnuts or pecans)
- Greek yogurt or low-fat whipped cream for serving (optional)

Prep Time: 10 minutes
Cook Time: 30 minutes
Instructions:
- Preheat the oven to 375°F (190°C).
- Place cored apples in a baking dish.
- Drizzle honey or maple syrup over the apples.
- Sprinkle ground cinnamon and chopped nuts over the apples.
- Bake for 25-30 minutes, or until the apples are tender.
- Serve warm, topped with Greek yogurt or low-fat whipped cream if desired.

Nutritional Values (per serving):
- Total Carbohydrate: 25g
- Dietary Fiber: 5g
- Total Sugars: 18g
- Protein: 2g
- Total Fat: 7g
- Saturated Fat: 1g
- Cholesterol: 0mg
- Vitamin A: 49IU
- Vitamin C: 8mg
- Folate: 3mcg
- Sodium: 2mg
- Calcium: 28mg
- Iron: 1mg
- Magnesium: 18mg
- Potassium: 195mg

COCONUT CHIA SEED PUDDING

Servings: 4
Ingredients:

- 1/4 cup chia seeds
- 1 cup coconut milk
- 1 tablespoon honey or maple syrup
- 1/2 teaspoon vanilla extract
- Toasted coconut flakes for topping

Prep Time: 5 minutes
Cook Time: 0 minutes
Instructions:

- In a mixing bowl, whisk together chia seeds, coconut milk, honey or maple syrup, and vanilla extract.
- Let the mixture sit for 5 minutes, then whisk again to prevent clumps.
- Cover the bowl and refrigerate for at least 2 hours, or overnight, until the chia pudding thickens.
- Stir the pudding before serving and divide into serving cups.
- Top with toasted coconut flakes.
- Serve chilled.

Nutritional Values (per serving):

- Total Carbohydrate: 7g
- Dietary Fiber: 4g
- Total Sugars: 3g
- Protein: 3g
- Total Fat: 16g
- Saturated Fat: 12g
- Cholesterol: 0mg
- Vitamin A: 0IU
- Vitamin C: 0mg
- Folate: 16mcg
- Sodium: 9mg
- Calcium: 82mg
- Iron: 2mg
- Magnesium: 80mg
- Potassium: 142mg

PUMPKIN SPICE BITES

Servings: 8
Ingredients:

- 1 cup rolled oats
- 1/2 cup canned pumpkin puree
- 1/4 cup almond butter
- 2 tablespoons honey or maple syrup
- 1 teaspoon pumpkin pie spice
- 1/4 cup dark chocolate chips (optional)

Prep Time: 10 minutes
Cook Time: 0 minutes
Instructions:

- In a mixing bowl, combine rolled oats, canned pumpkin puree, almond butter, honey or maple syrup, and pumpkin pie spice.
- Fold in dark chocolate chips if using.
- Roll the mixture into bite-sized balls using your hands.
- Place the balls on a baking sheet lined with parchment paper.
- Refrigerate for at least 30 minutes to firm up.
- Serve chilled.

Nutritional Values (per serving):

- Total Carbohydrate: 14g
- Dietary Fiber: 2g
- Total Sugars: 6g
- Protein: 3g
- Total Fat: 6g
- Saturated Fat: 1g
- Cholesterol: 0mg
- Vitamin A: 2393IU
- Vitamin C: 1mg
- Folate: 8mcg
- Sodium: 2mg
- Calcium: 22mg
- Iron: 1mg
- Magnesium: 32mg
- Potassium: 102mg

MIXED BERRY SORBET

Servings: 4
Ingredients:
- 2 cups mixed berries (such as strawberries, blueberries, raspberries)
- 1 tablespoon lemon juice
- 2 tablespoons honey or maple syrup
- Fresh mint leaves for garnish (optional)

Prep Time: 5 minutes
Cook Time: 0 minutes
Instructions:
- In a blender or food processor, combine mixed berries, lemon juice, and honey or maple syrup.
- Blend until smooth.
- Pour the mixture into a shallow dish and freeze for 3-4 hours, or until firm.
- Remove from the freezer and let sit at room temperature for 5 minutes before scooping.
- Garnish with fresh mint leaves if desired.
- Serve immediately.

Nutritional Values (per serving):
- Total Carbohydrate: 19g
- Dietary Fiber: 4g
- Total Sugars: 14g
- Protein: 1g
- Total Fat: 0g
- Saturated Fat: 0g
- Cholesterol: 0mg
- Vitamin A: 121IU
- Vitamin C: 25mg
- Folate: 19mcg
- Sodium: 1mg
- Calcium: 16mg
- Iron: 0mg
- Magnesium: 15mg
- Potassium: 147mg

LEMON COCONUT BLISS BALLS

Servings: 8
Ingredients:
- 1 cup unsweetened shredded coconut
- 1/4 cup almond flour
- 2 tablespoons honey or maple syrup
- Zest and juice of 1 lemon
- 1/2 teaspoon vanilla extract

Prep Time: 10 minutes
Cook Time: 0 minutes
Instructions:
- In a food processor, combine unsweetened shredded coconut, almond flour, honey or maple syrup, lemon zest, lemon juice, and vanilla extract.
- Process until the mixture comes together and sticks together when pressed between your fingers.
- Roll the mixture into bite-sized balls using your hands.
- Place the balls on a baking sheet lined with parchment paper.
- Refrigerate for at least 30 minutes to firm up.
- Serve chilled.

Nutritional Values (per serving):
- Total Carbohydrate: 6g
- Dietary Fiber: 2g
- Total Sugars: 3g
- Protein: 1g
- Total Fat: 6g
- Saturated Fat: 5g
- Cholesterol: 0mg
- Vitamin A: 0IU
- Vitamin C: 2mg
- Folate: 4mcg
- Sodium: 3mg
- Calcium: 7mg
- Iron: 0mg
- Magnesium: 10mg
- Potassium: 51mg

PEANUT BUTTER BANANA OAT COOKIES

Servings: 12 cookies
Ingredients:
- 2 ripe bananas, mashed
- 1/2 cup creamy peanut butter
- 1 cup rolled oats
- 1/4 cup chopped walnuts
- 1/4 cup dark chocolate chips (optional)

Prep Time: 10 minutes
Cook Time: 15 minutes
Instructions:
- Preheat the oven to 350°F (175°C). Line a baking sheet with parchment paper.
- In a mixing bowl, combine mashed bananas, creamy peanut butter, rolled oats, chopped walnuts, and dark chocolate chips (if using). Mix until well combined.
- Scoop spoonfuls of the dough onto the prepared baking sheet, spacing them apart.
- Use a fork to flatten each cookie slightly.
- Bake for 12-15 minutes, or until the cookies are golden brown around the edges.
- Remove from the oven and let cool on the baking sheet for 5 minutes before transferring to a wire rack to cool completely.
- Store leftovers in an airtight container at room temperature for up to 3 days.

Nutritional Values (per serving - 1 cookie):
- Total Carbohydrate: 13g
- Dietary Fiber: 2g
- Total Sugars: 5g
- Protein: 4g
- Total Fat: 8g
- Saturated Fat: 2g
- Cholesterol: 0mg
- Vitamin A: 11IU
- Vitamin C: 1mg
- Folate: 15mcg
- Sodium: 50mg
- Calcium: 13mg
- Iron: 1mg
- Magnesium: 34mg
- Potassium: 170mg

CHAPTER 10: MEASUREMENT CHART

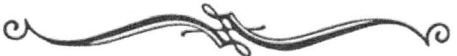

Ingredient	Measurement
Flour	1 cup
Sugar	1 tablespoon
Brown Sugar	1 tablespoon
Butter	1 tablespoon
Olive Oil	1 tablespoon
Milk	1 cup
Yogurt	1/2 cup
Honey	1 tablespoon
Maple Syrup	1 tablespoon
Baking Powder	1 teaspoon
Baking Soda	1/2 teaspoon
Salt	1/4 teaspoon
Cinnamon	1 teaspoon
Nutmeg	1/4 teaspoon
Vanilla Extract	1 teaspoon
Lemon Juice	1 tablespoon
Vinegar	1 tablespoon
Cocoa Powder	2 tablespoons
Coconut Milk	1 cup
Almond Flour	1/4 cup
Chia Seeds	2 tablespoons
Rolled Oats	1 cup
Shredded Coconut	1/2 cup
Almond Butter	1/4 cup
Walnuts	1/4 cup
Pecans	1/4 cup
Sesame Seeds	2 tablespoons
Rice Vinegar	2 tablespoons

4-WEEK MEAL PLAN

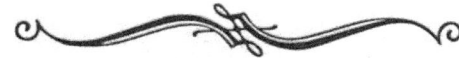

Week 1:

Day	Breakfast	Lunch	Dinner	Snack
Monday	Veggie Omelette	Greek Chicken Salad	Baked Salmon with Roasted Vegetables	Apple Slices with Almond Butter
Tuesday	Berry Smoothie Bowl	Quinoa Salad with Chickpeas	Turkey Meatballs with Zucchini Noodles	Carrot Sticks with Hummus
Wednesday	Greek Yogurt Parfait with Granola	Lentil Soup	Grilled Chicken with Steamed Broccoli	Mixed Nuts
Thursday	Whole Wheat Pancakes with Berries	Tuna Salad Lettuce Wraps	Eggplant Parmesan with Mixed Greens Salad	Cottage Cheese with Pineapple
Friday	Avocado Toast with Poached Eggs	Caprese Salad with Balsamic Glaze	Beef Stir-Fry with Brown Rice	Greek Yogurt with Mixed Berries
Saturday	Chia Seed Pudding with Fresh Fruit	Quinoa Stuffed Bell Peppers	Grilled Shrimp Skewers with Quinoa Salad	Cucumber Slices with Guacamole
Sunday	Banana Oatmeal Muffins	Mediterranean Chickpea Salad	Vegetable Stir-Fry with Tofu	Rice Cakes with Peanut Butter

Week 2:

Day	Breakfast	Lunch	Dinner	Snack
Monday	Scrambled Eggs with Spinach	Turkey and Avocado Wrap	Grilled Salmon with Asparagus	Bell Pepper Slices with Hummus
Tuesday	Green Smoothie	Quinoa and Black Bean Salad	Chicken Fajitas with Whole Wheat Tortillas	Greek Yogurt with Granola
Wednesday	Cottage Cheese with Berries	Lentil and Vegetable Soup	Baked Chicken Parmesan with Zucchini Noodles	Almonds

Thursday	Banana Pancakes	Tofu and Vegetable Stir-Fry	Shrimp and Vegetable Skewers with Brown Rice	Carrot Sticks with Almond Butter
Friday	Yogurt Parfait with Mixed Berries	Chickpea and Avocado Salad	Beef and Broccoli Stir-Fry with Quinoa	Apple Slices with Peanut Butter
Saturday	Oatmeal with Sliced Banana	Greek Salad with Grilled Chicken	Eggplant and Tomato Bake	Celery Sticks with Cream Cheese
Sunday	Breakfast Burrito	Lentil and Quinoa Salad	Turkey Meatloaf with Mashed Cauliflower	Cheese and Whole Grain Crackers

Week 3:

Day	Breakfast	Lunch	Dinner	Snack
Monday	Blueberry Muffins	Spinach and Feta Salad	Baked Cod with Roasted Vegetables	Trail Mix
Tuesday	Chia Seed Pudding with Mango	Chicken and Vegetable Stir-Fry	Spaghetti Squash with Turkey Bolognese	Orange Slices
Wednesday	Peanut Butter Banana Smoothie Bowl	Greek Salad with Tuna	Grilled Steak with Garlic Green Beans	Hard-boiled Eggs
Thursday	Whole Wheat Waffles with Strawberries	Lentil Soup	Stuffed Bell Peppers	Cheese Slices
Friday	Breakfast Quesadilla	Turkey and Quinoa Salad	Lemon Herb Chicken with Steamed Broccoli	Rice Cakes with Avocado
Saturday	Yogurt Bowl with Almonds and Berries	Mediterranean Couscous Salad	Shrimp Scampi with Whole Wheat Pasta	Tomato Slices with Basil
Sunday	Breakfast Casserole	Caprese Stuffed Portobello Mushrooms	Baked Chicken with Sweet Potato Mash	Greek Yogurt with Honey

Week 4:

Day	Breakfast	Lunch	Dinner	Snack
Monday	Vegetable Frittata	Chickpea Salad	Grilled Swordfish with Quinoa Salad	Bell Pepper Slices with Hummus
Tuesday	Smoothie Bowl with Mixed Berries	Turkey Lettuce Wraps	Eggplant Rollatini with Side Salad	Almonds
Wednesday	Overnight Oats with Peanut Butter	Greek Salad with Grilled Chicken	Baked Salmon with Steamed Vegetables	Carrot Sticks with Almond Butter
Thursday	Breakfast Burrito	Lentil Soup	Turkey Chili with Cauliflower Rice	Greek Yogurt with Granola
Friday	Banana Pancakes	Tuna Salad Sandwich	Beef Stir-Fry with Brown Rice	Apple Slices with Peanut Butter
Saturday	Avocado Toast with Poached Eggs	Quinoa and Black Bean Salad	Chicken Piccata with Asparagus	Cheese and Whole Grain Crackers
Sunday	Omelette with Spinach and Mushrooms	Lentil and Vegetable Soup	Baked Cod with Roasted Brussels Sprouts	Trail Mix

BONUS SECTION:
COOKING TIPS AND TECHNIQUES

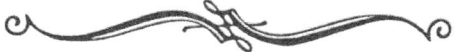

In this section, we delve into essential cooking tips and techniques to help you prepare delicious and nutritious meals while maintaining a healthy lifestyle. We'll explore healthier cooking methods, ways to flavor foods without excess sugar and salt, and provide insights into optimizing your culinary skills.

1. Healthier Cooking Methods:

Grilling: Grilling is a fantastic way to add flavor to your meals without the need for excessive oil or added fats. Whether it's vegetables, lean meats, or seafood, grilling imparts a delicious smoky flavor while allowing excess fats to drip away.

Baking and Roasting: Baking and roasting are excellent methods for cooking a wide variety of foods, from vegetables to proteins. By using the oven, you can cook foods with minimal added fats while retaining their natural flavors and nutrients.

Steaming: Steaming is a gentle cooking method that preserves the nutritional content of foods while imparting a subtle, delicate flavor. It's perfect for vegetables, fish, and even grains like rice and quinoa.

Stir-Frying: Stir-frying involves quickly cooking small pieces of food in a small amount of oil over high heat. This method retains the vibrant colors and crisp textures of vegetables while requiring minimal oil.

Poaching: Poaching involves cooking foods gently in simmering liquid, such as water or broth. It's an excellent method for cooking delicate proteins like fish or eggs without adding excess fats.

2. Flavoring Foods without Excess Sugar and Salt:

Herbs and Spices: Herbs and spices are nature's flavor enhancers, offering a wide range of tastes without the need for added sugar or salt. Experiment with aromatic herbs like basil, thyme, and rosemary, as well as spices like cumin, paprika, and turmeric to add depth and complexity to your dishes.

Citrus Zest and Juice: Citrus zest and juice provide a burst of bright, tangy flavor to your meals without adding extra calories or sodium. Use lemon, lime, or orange zest to add zing to salads, marinades, and dressings.

Vinegars: Vinegars, such as balsamic, apple cider, or rice vinegar, can add acidity and depth to dishes without the need for salt. Drizzle a splash of vinegar over roasted vegetables or use it to deglaze pans for sauces and marinades.

Umami-rich Ingredients: **Ingredients like mushrooms, tomatoes, and soy sauce are naturally rich in umami, the savory fifth taste. Incorporate these ingredients into your recipes to enhance flavor without relying on salt or sugar.**

Homemade Seasoning Blends: Create your own seasoning blends using a combination of herbs, spices, and aromatics. Experiment with different flavor profiles, such as Mediterranean, Mexican, or Asian-inspired blends, to keep your meals exciting and flavorful.

3. Additional Tips and Insights:

Use High-Quality Ingredients: **Opt for fresh, high-quality ingredients whenever possible to elevate the flavor of your dishes naturally.**

Experiment with Healthy Fats: Incorporate healthy fats like olive oil, avocado, and nuts into your cooking to add richness and depth of flavor without compromising on nutrition.

Balance Flavors: Aim for a balance of sweet, salty, sour, and savory flavors in your dishes to create a well-rounded and satisfying culinary experience.

Mindful Seasoning: Taste your food as you cook and adjust seasoning gradually to avoid overdoing it with salt or sugar. Remember, you can always add more seasoning, but it's challenging to remove excess once it's added.

Explore Global Cuisine: Embrace the diverse flavors of world cuisine by exploring recipes from different cultures. You'll discover new ingredients and techniques that can inspire healthy and flavorful cooking.

CONCLUSION

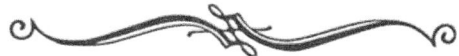

Congratulations on embarking on your journey to healthier eating with "The Comprehensive Diabetic Diet After 50" cookbook! As you've navigated through the pages of this book, you've gained valuable insights into managing your diabetes through delicious, nutritious, and diabetes-friendly recipes.

In this concluding chapter, let's reflect on the key takeaways and actionable steps you can implement to optimize your health and well-being:

1. Knowledge is Power:

- Understanding the fundamentals of diabetes, including its causes, symptoms, and risk factors, empowers you to take control of your health.
- By learning about the role of insulin, the importance of early detection, and diagnostic tests, you can proactively manage your diabetes and make informed decisions about your lifestyle and dietary choices.

2. Embracing Healthy Eating Habits:

- Adopting a balanced and diverse diet rich in whole grains, lean proteins, healthy fats, and plenty of fruits and vegetables is essential for managing diabetes and promoting overall wellness.
- Experimenting with new recipes and incorporating flavorful herbs, spices, and seasoning blends allows you to enjoy delicious meals without relying on excess sugar or salt.

3. Cooking with Confidence:

- Equipping yourself with cooking tips and techniques, such as grilling, baking, and flavoring foods with natural ingredients, empowers you to prepare nutritious and satisfying meals at home.
- By embracing healthier cooking methods and mindful seasoning practices, you can unleash your culinary creativity and transform everyday meals into culinary delights.

4. Cultivating a Positive Mindset:

- Diabetes management is not just about physical health but also about nurturing a positive mindset and emotional well-being.
- Celebrate your successes, no matter how small, and acknowledge the progress you've made towards your health goals. Remember that every step you take towards a healthier lifestyle is a step in the right direction.

5. Community and Support:

- Surrounding yourself with a supportive network of family, friends, and healthcare professionals can provide encouragement, accountability, and motivation on your journey.
- Share your experiences, challenges, and successes with others who understand and empathize with your journey towards better health.

3 BONUSES FOR YOU!

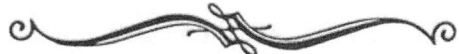

As a special thank you for joining us on this journey, we're thrilled to offer you access to exclusive bonus content. Simply scan the QR code below using your smartphone or tablet or email thomasdharman4@gmail.com (indicating "BONUS DIABETIC" as the subject line) to download these valuable resources in PDF format:

Upon scanning the QR code, you'll unlock access to the following bonus materials:

BONUS #1: Guide to Foods and Portions for Diabetics

Discover a comprehensive guide packed with essential information on foods tailored for managing diabetes. From foods to prioritize to those best avoided, this guide will empower you to make informed choices about your diet. You'll also find a handy table outlining recommended portions for various food categories, ensuring you maintain optimal control over your diet.

BONUS #2: Guide to Healthy Shopping

Transform your grocery shopping experience with this invaluable guide to healthy eating. Learn how to decipher food labels to identify hidden sugars, saturated fats, sodium, and more. We'll also provide you with a curated list of staple foods that should be in every diabetic's pantry. Plus, gain insider tips for saving time and money while grocery shopping without compromising on the quality of your diet.

BONUS #3: Checklist for Traveling with Diabetes

Embark on your next adventure with confidence using our comprehensive checklist for traveling with diabetes. From packing essential supplies to managing meals away from home, this resource is your go-to companion for stress-free travel. Say goodbye to travel worries and hello to seamless journeys!

As you close the pages of "The Comprehensive Diabetic Diet After 50," remember that your health is your greatest asset, and investing in it through mindful nutrition and lifestyle choices is a lifelong commitment. Embrace the journey with curiosity, resilience, and determination, knowing that you have the knowledge, skills, and resources to thrive with diabetes and live your best life.

Here's to your continued health, happiness, and vitality!

Warmest regards,

Thomas Dharman

Made in the USA
Monee, IL
04 August 2024